intro*duction*

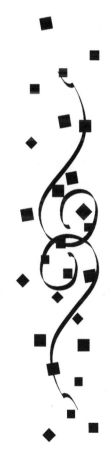

Printed in the United States of America

Book design and layout by Ecoversity, Manvel, TX

Printed by Met Printing, Houston, TX

ISBN 0-9659359-1-4

Ah, Desserts. Sweets. Chocolate. Bad words when you're a diabetic. Now it doesn't have to be. This cookbook is written solely with the diabetic in mind to enjoy those off-limits treats. Well, off-limits no more! Enjoy recipes like Almond Meringue Torte and Chocolate Chips Oatmeal Cookies without too much worry. By using ingredients like maltitol, you can enjoy the sweets without the usual raise in blood sugar. So have that dessert after dinner. Relax in the morning with a slice of coffee cake. Celebrate that promotion or special event with a slice of cheesecake. But, as with all sweets, moderation is the key.

Enjoy!
Mary Halmon

A book would not be complete without a few thank yous...

... To Amy Ludzig, chef and great typist, thank you for being "Recipe Editor" and assistant, and for all your hard work.

... To Dr. Louis Train, Sr., M.D., thank you for all your help, research and support on finding an alternative ingredient to make a diabetic's life so much easier.

... And to Virginia and George Uppencamp who were most instrumental in inspiring me to create a diabetic cookbook and encouraged me to look for something new. Without your inspiration, this book would never have happened. Your help and friendship means a lot to me and I thank you from the bottom of my heart.

...To Gary and Donna Cowart, thanks for all the help you have done for me with electrical work and kindness to my husband. Donna has always been so kind to us every time I called and needed something, she got Gary to come and fix it! God Bless You Both.

... To Allen Williams at Randalls on Holcombe at Buffalo Speedway, thank you for your kindness and help time and time again.

... To Joe at La Madeleine French Bakery & Cafe in the Village, thank you so much for everything. You've been extremely helpful, kind and supportive.

... And to all the vendors who have supported this project and sent samples. A big Texas thank you!

If I have forgotten someone, I apologize, but your support is greatly appreciated.

Equivalents for Sugar Substitutions

Brand Name		Equivalent Amount of Sugar
Adolph's (powder)		
2 shakes of jar	=	1 rounded teaspoon sugar
1/4 teaspoon	=	1 tablespoon
1 teaspoon	=	1/4 cup
2 1/2 teaspoons	=	2/3 cup
1 tablespoon	=	3/4 cup
4 teaspoons	=	1 cup
Equal (powder)*		
1 packet	=	2 teaspoons
Fasweet (liquid)		
1/8 teaspoon	=	1 teaspoon
1/4 teaspoon	=	2 teaspoon
1/3 teaspoon	=	1 tablespoon
1 tablespoon	=	1/2 cup
2 tablespoons	=	1 cup
Maltitol (Steel's Nature Sweet, liquid)		
1 teaspoon	=	1 teaspoon
Sucaryl (liquid)		
1/8 teaspoon	=	1 teaspoon
1/3 teaspoon	=	1 tablespoon
1/2 teaspoon	=	4 teaspoons
1 1/2 teaspoons	=	1/4 cup
1 tablespoons	=	1/2 cup

Superose (liquid)

4 drops	=	1 teaspoon
1/8 teaspoon	=	2 teaspoon
1/4 teaspoon plus 4 drops	=	1 tablespoon
1 1/2 teaspoons	=	1/2 cup
1 tablespoon	=	1 cup

Sugar Twin (powder)

1 teaspoon	=	1 teaspoon

Sugar Twin, Brown (powder)

1 teaspoon	=	1 teaspoon brown

Sweet N' Low (powder)

1/10 teaspoon	=	1 teaspoon
1 packet	=	2 teaspoon
1/3 teaspoon	=	1 tablespoon
1 teaspoon	=	1/4 cup
1 1/4 teaspoons	=	1/3 cup
2 teaspoons	=	1/2 cup
4 teaspoons	=	1 cup

Sweet N' Low, Brown (powder)

1/4 teaspoon	=	1 tablespoon
1 teaspoon	=	1/4 cup
1 1/3 teaspoons	=	1/3 cup
2 teaspoons	=	1/2 cup
4 teaspoons	=	1 cup

Sweet'ner (powder)

1 packet	=	2 teaspoons

Sweet Majic (powder)

1 packet	=	2 teaspoons

Sweet One (powder)

1 packet	=	2 teaspoons
3 packets	=	1/4 cup
4 packets	=	1/3 cup
6 packets	=	1/2 cup
12 packets	=	1 cup

Sweet-10 (liquid)

10 drops	=	1 teaspoon
1/2 teaspoon	=	4 teaspoons
1 1/2 teaspoons	=	1/4 cup
1 tablespoon	=	1/2 cup
2 tablespoon	=	1 cup

Zero-Cal (liquid)

10 drops	=	1 teaspoon
30 drops	=	1 tablespoon
3/4 teaspoon	=	2 tablespoons
1 tablespoon	=	1/2 cup
2 tablespoons	=	1 cup

*Use only after cooking or in uncooked dishes

breakfast
sweets

Acorn Squash Coffee Cake

Serving Size: 9

1/4 cup soft butter
1/4 cup brown sugar replacement
1/2 cup maltitol
1 large egg
1 cup cooked and mashed acorn squash
2 cups all-purpose flour
2 tsps baking soda
1 tsp cinnamon
1/2 tsp salt
1 cup chopped pecans
Topping:
1/2 cup brown sugar replacement
1/3 cup all-purpose flour
1/2 tsp cinnamon
1/4 cup soft butter
1/2 cup chopped pecans

Preheat oven to 350°F and spray a 9 inch square baking dish with nonstick cooking spray, set aside. Whip butter until light and fluffy then gradually add brown sugar replacement and maltitol. Add egg, mix well. Stir in squash. Combine remaining ingredients and gradually add to squash mixture. Pour batter into pan and top with streusel mixture. Bake for 40 minutes. Serve warm.

Streusel mixture: Combine all ingredients and stir well.

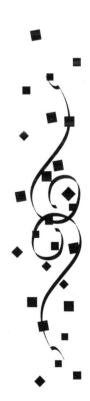

Apple Coffee Cake

Serving Size: 9

3/4 cup milk
1 package yeast
1/4 cup water
3 1/4 cups all-purpose flour
2 eggs
1/2 cup soft butter
1/2 cup maltitol
1/2 tsp salt
2 tbsps melted butter, cooled
1 tbsp brown sugar replacement
3 cups apple slices
1/2 tsp ground cinnamon
1/8 tsp ground nutmeg
1/2 cup brown sugar replacement

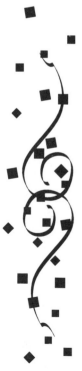

Preheat oven to 375°F. Spray a 9 inch square baking dish with nonstick cooking spray, set aside. Scald milk; cool to lukewarm. Dissolve yeast in warm water. Add the cooled milk. Stir in 1-1/2 cups flour; beat until smooth. Cover and let rise until doubled in size, about 1 hour. Punch down and add eggs, one at a time, beating well after each. Stir in 1/2 cup butter, 1/2 cup maltitol, salt and the remaining flour. Beat well. Spread the dough in the prepared baking pan. Spoon 2 tablespoons butter and 1 tablespoon brown sugar replacement over dough. Cover; let rise until double. Press apples into dough. Mix cinnamon, nutmeg and 1/2 cup brown sugar replacement. Sprinkle over fruit. Bake for 40-45 minutes.

Banana Pecan Coffee Cake

Serving size: 12

1 cup maltitol
2 sticks margarine, melted
1/4 cup skim milk
2 egg whites
1 tsp vanilla
2-4 mashed bananas
2 cups flour
1 tsp baking soda
Topping
1 stick margarine, melted
1 cup brown sugar replacement
1 cup chopped pecans

Preheat oven to 350°F. Prepare a 9x13 inch pan with nonstick cooking spray. Mix maltitol, 2 sticks melted margarine, milk, egg whites, vanilla, bananas, flour and soda. Pour into prepared pan. Mix topping ingredients together. Pour over top of cake. Bake 30 to 40 minutes or until done.

Quick Hints
Too High Low Flame?
If adjusting the flame on your gas stove low enough to maintain a slow simmer proves to troublesome, try this: Place two burner grates one on top of the other. By elevating the pan above the flame, this gives you the equivalent of a very low flame, great for simmering.

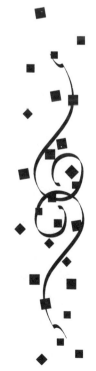

Chocolate Waffles

Serving Size: 4

1 1/2 cups flour
1/4 cup unsweetened cocoa powder
1 tsp baking powder
1 tsp baking soda
1/3 cup maltitol
2 cups lowfat buttermilk
1/2 cup canola oil
2 large eggs, separated
1 tsp vanilla extract
Pinch cream of tartar

Sift together flour, cocoa, baking powder and baking soda.
Make a well in center of sifted dry ingredients. In a separate
bowl mix maltitol, buttermilk, oil, egg yolks, and vanilla. Pour
into the well and mix with dry ingredients. Beat egg whites
with cream of tartar until soft peaks form. Gradually fold into
batter, one third at a time. Cook in waffle iron according to
manufacturer's instructions.

Serving Ideas: Serve with sweetened whipped cream or a
dessert sauce.

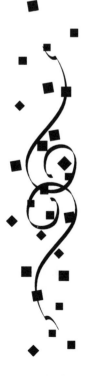

Cinnamon French Toast

Serving Size: 8

1 1/2 cups egg substitute
1/3 cup orange juice
1/3 cup skim milk
3 tbsp maltitol
1 tbsp orange zest, chopped
1 tbsp vanilla
2 tsp cinnamon
1 loaf French bread, 1 1/2 inch thick slices
Corn oil margarine or butter
Topping of choice

Beat egg substitute, orange juice, milk, maltitol, zest, vanilla
and cinnamon in bowl. Whisk until blended. Place bread in a
shallow baking dish in a single layer. Pour egg mixture over
bread. Let stand until saturated about 30 minutes, turning
once. Heat skillet to medium-high, add 3 tablespoons
margarine. Saute bread slices, turning once until golden
brown. Cook 2 minutes on each side. To serve, arrange on
serving platter. Top with favorite sugarfree topping.

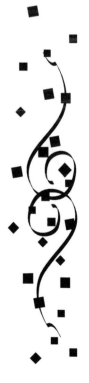

Hazelnut Coffee Cake

Serving Size: 10

1 recipe nut cake made with hazelnuts
1/2 cup hazelnut liqueur
1 recipe coffee buttercream
 chopped hazelnuts, toasted

Place one cake layer on cake plate and soak with 1/4 cup of hazelnut liqueur. Spread frosting over top. Put other layer on top and soak with remaining liqueur. Spread top and sided of cake with frosting and sprinkle the cake with chopped hazelnuts, if desired.

Notes: This recipe can be used for an almond coffee cake if you replace the hazelnuts with almonds and use amaretto to soak the cake.

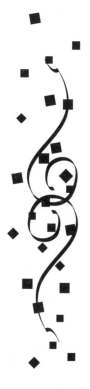

Overnight Oatmeal Waffles

Serving Size: 3

1/2 cup water
1 package dry yeast
2 cups skim milk, warmed
1/2 cup butter or margarine, melted
1 tsp salt
1 tsp maltitol
1 3/4 cup all purpose flour
1/4 cup whole wheat flour
1/3 cup regular oats

Next morning:
1 egg
1 egg white
1/4 tsp baking soda

The night before: Dissolve yeast in water for 5 minutes. Add milk, butter, salt, maltitol, flour and oats. Mix until smooth. Cover and stand overnight.

The next morning: Beat eggs and baking soda into batter until well mixed. Batter will be thin. Cook in waffle iron according to manufacturer's instructions.

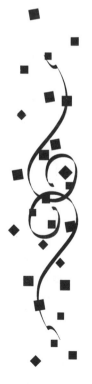

Plum and Sour Cream Coffee Cake

Serving Size: 12

1 cup butter at room temperature
1 1/4 cups maltitol
2 eggs
1 cup sour cream
1 1/2 tsps vanilla extract
2 cups all-purpose flour
1 tsp baking powder
1/2 tsp baking soda
1/4 tsp salt
1 cup plums, pitted and chopped
Topping
1 1/4 cups sliced almonds
1/4 cup brown sugar replacement
2 tsps ground cinnamon

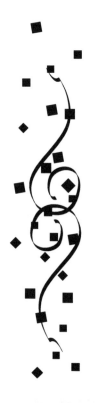

Preheat oven to 350°F and spray a 9-inch tube pan with nonstick cooking spray. In large bowl of electric mixer, cream butter and maltitol until light and fluffy. Beat in eggs, sour cream, and vanilla. Stir together flour, baking powder, baking soda, and salt. Gradually beat into butter mixture. Fold in plums. In a small bowl, combine nuts, sugar, and cinnamon for topping. Scatter half the topping evenly over bottom of pan. Spoon in half the batter. Add remaining topping and spoon on remaining batter. Bake 50 to 60 minutes, or until toothpick inserted in center comes out clean. Cool 15 minutes before removing from pan.

Rhubarb Coffee Cake

Serving Size: 8

Filling
4 cups rhubarb (about 8 stalks), do not use leaves
1/2 cup sugar
1/4 cup flour
2 tbsps butter
2 tsps ground cinnamon
Batter
3/4 cup butter
1 cup sugar
2 eggs
1 tsp vanilla extract
2 cups all-purpose flour
1 tsp baking powder
1/4 tsp baking soda
1 pinch salt
 grated peel of 1 lemon
1 cup nonfat sour cream
Topping
1/4 cup butter
1/2 cup brown sugar replacement
1 tsp ground cinnamon
1/2 cup flour

Preheat oven to 400°F and spray a 9-inch springform pan with nonstick cooking spray. To make filling: Wash and dry rhubarb stalks. Slice into 1-inch pieces and place in a medium bowl. Toss with maltitol, flour, butter, and cinnamon. Set aside.

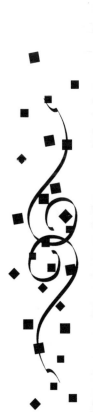

continued on page 20

To make batter: In a large mixing bowl, beat butter and maltitol together until light and fluffy. Beat in eggs and vanilla. Sift flour, baking powder, baking soda, and salt. Stir lemon peel into sour cream. Fold half of sifted flour mixture into butter-sugar-egg mixture. Fold in sour cream-lemon peel. Fold in remaining flour. Mix well.

To make topping: In a small bowl, mix butter, brown sugar replacement, and cinnamon. Mix in flour until crumbly. Place half the batter in prepared pan. Cover batter with filling. Top with remaining batter. Sprinkle on topping. Bake for 1 hour and 10 minutes. Cool in pan 10 minutes; carefully remove pan sides; cool completely on wire rack.

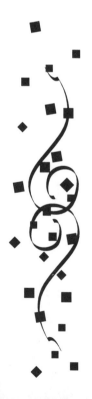

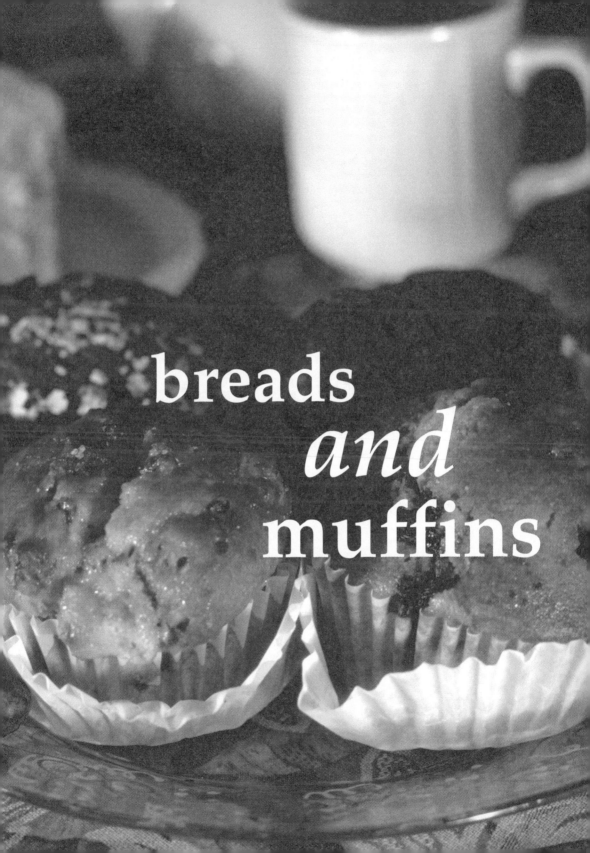

breads *and* muffins

Apple Banana Bread

Serving Size: 10

1/2 cup butter, softened
1/2 cup brown sugar substitute
1/2 cup maltitol
2 eggs
3 tbsps sour cream
1/2 cup mashed bananas (2 bananas)
1 tsp vanilla extract
2 cups all-purpose flour
1 tsp baking powder
1 tsp baking soda
1/2 tsp ground cinnamon
2 medium Golden delicious apples, chopped
1/2 cup chopped pecans

Preheat oven to 375°F and spray a 9x5x3 inch loaf pan
with nonstick cooking spray, set aside. Cream together
butter and brown sugar replacement, then gradually add
in maltitol. Beat in eggs, one at a time, beating thoroughly
after each addition. Blend in sour cream, banana and
vanilla. Combine flour, baking powder, soda and
cinnamon. Gradually add to butter mixture. Gently fold in
chopped apples and pecans. Pour into loaf pan. Bake
about 1 hour. Cool 10 minutes in pan before turning out
onto a rack to cool completely before slicing.

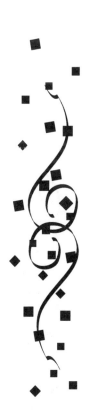

Apple Pecan Bread

Serving Size: 10

1/2 cup canola oil
3/4 cup maltitol
2 eggs
2 cups all-purpose flour
1 tsp baking powder
1 tsp baking soda
1 cup Granny Smith apples, cored and diced
1/2 cup chopped pecans

Preheat oven to 350°F and spray a 9X5X3 inch loaf pan with nonstick cooking spray, set aside. Combine oil, maltitol and eggs. Add flour, baking powder, and soda and stir just until blended. Stir in apples and nuts, then pour into prepared pan. Bake for one hour or until a knife inserted in the center comes out clean. Remove from pan and cool on a rack. This bread is best if wrapped overnight and eaten the next day.

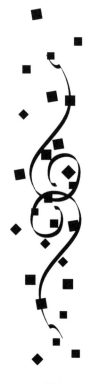

Applesauce Raisin Nut Bread

Serving Size: 10

1 1/2 cups whole-wheat flour
3 tsps baking powder
1 tsp salt
1 tsp cinnamon
1/2 tsp nutmeg
1 cup oats
1/2 cup maltitol
2 whole eggs, lightly beaten
1/3 cup salad oil
1 cup applesauce
1/2 cup raisins soaked in hot water
1/2 cup pecans

Preheat oven to 350°F and spray a 9X5X3 inch loaf pan with nonstick cooking spray. Sift together flour, baking powder, salt, cinnamon, and nutmeg. Stir in oats and maltitol. Blend eggs, oil and applesauce together. Stir in dry ingredients, raisins and nuts. Pour into loaf pan. Bake for 1 hour or until a knife inserted in the middle of the loaf comes out clean. Allow bread to cool 10 minutes in pan before turning out onto a rack to finish cooling.

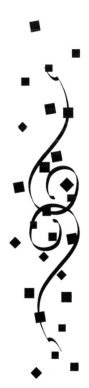

Banana Nut Bread

Serving Size: 10

3/4 cup butter
1 1/2 cups maltitol
1 1/2 cups mashed bananas
2 eggs
1 tsp vanilla extract
2 cups all-purpose flour
1 tsp baking soda
3/4 tsp salt
1/2 cup buttermilk
3/4 cup pecans, chopped

Preheat oven to 350°F and spray a 9X5X3 inch loaf pan with nonstick cooking spray. Cream together butter and maltitol. Add banana, eggs, and vanilla. Sift together dry ingredients. Add alternately with buttermilk. Blend well. Stir in pecans, and pour into prepared loaf pan. Bake 1-1/4 hours or until a knife inserted in the middle of the loaf comes out clean. Allow to cool 10 minutes in pan before turning out onto a rack to finish cooling.

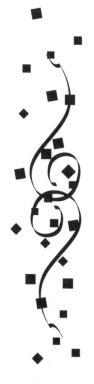

Blueberry Quick Bread

Serving Size: 10

2 tbsps sifted cake flour
2 tbsps brown sugar replacement
1/2 tsp cinnamon
1 tbsp chopped almonds
1/2 cup butter, divided
1 1/2 cups blueberries
3 cups sifted cake flour, divided
2 tsps baking powder
1 1/2 cups maltitol
1 large egg, lightly beaten
1 cup milk

Preheat oven to 350°F and spray a 9X5X3 inch loaf pan with nonstick cooking spray, set aside. Combine first 4 ingredients and add 1 teaspoon of butter, stir until crumbly, set aside. Combine blueberries with 2 tablespoons flour, set aside. Combine remaining flour, baking powder and salt, and cut in remaining butter until crumbly. Combine maltitol, egg and milk, stir well. Add egg mixture to flour mixture and stir just until the dry ingredients are moistened. Gently fold in blueberries. Pour batter into prepared pan, sprinkle top with almond mixture, and bake 1 hour and 10 minutes or until a knife inserted in the center comes out clean. Cool in pan 10 minutes before removing to a rack to cool completely.

Notes: Fresh or frozen blueberries may be used in this recipe, but if you are using frozen blueberries, make sure they are not sweetened. Coating the berries in flour keeps them suspended in the bread and also keeps them from bleeding in the batter.

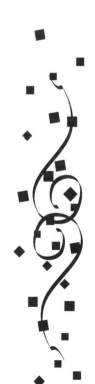

Brioche Rolls

Serving Size: 12

1/2 cup milk
1 envelope dry yeast
3/4 cup all-purpose flour, unbleached
6 tbsps unsalted butter, softened
3 tbsps maltitol
1/2 tsp salt
1 large egg
2 egg yolks
1 cup all-purpose flour, unbleached

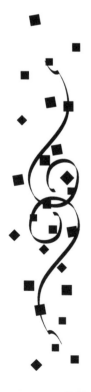

Heat the milk just until it feels warm, remove from heat. Place the milk in a bowl, and sprinkle yeast over it, and whisk until all yeast is dissolved. Add the first amount of flour, stir until incorporated. Cover the bowl with plastic wrap and let it sit at room temperature until it has at least doubled its size. While the first part of the dough is rising, start on the second half. Place the butter in a bowl and whip it until it is soft and almost white. While mixing, add the maltitol and salt and the egg and beat until smooth. Mix in 1/3 of the flour until it is absorbed. Add an egg yolk, and beat until it is absorbed. Mix in another 1/3 of the flour, then the last yolk. Add the first dough mixture if it has doubled its size at this time. Beat until the dough is smooth and very elastic, about 5 more minutes. Cover the completed dough with plastic wrap and allow the dough to double in size - about 1 hour. Remove the dough and deflate it by kneading it for a few minutes. Place the dough into a bowl that has been buttered and turn it over to butter all sides of the dough. Cover the bowl tightly and refrigerate for 2-3 hours, until it has risen again. Remove the dough from the refrigerator and deflate it again. Roll the dough into a thick rope and cut it into 12 even pieces. Roll the

continued on page 29

pieces of dough into 12 balls or ovals and place on a baking sheet that has been sprayed with nonstick cooking spray. Allow rolls to double in size, once more, and then brush the tops of the rolls with an egg that has been slightly beaten. Preheat oven to 350°F and bake 20 minutes, or until the rolls are a deep golden color. Remove the rolls from the pan so the can cool completely on a rack.

Notes: This bread is a little tedious to make, but I assure you it will be one of the most heavenly breads you have ever had!

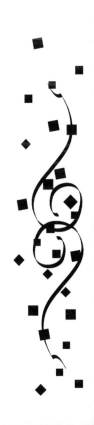

Challah Bread

Serving Size: 12

5 cups all-purpose flour, unbleached
1/3 cup maltitol
2 tsps salt
1 cup warm water
1 envelope dry yeast
1/4 cup canola oil
2 large eggs
1 egg yolk

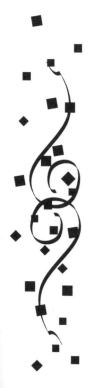

Combine water and yeast and set aside for five minutes. Stir yeast mixture until all yeast is dissolved and add to it maltitol, eggs and egg yolk, whisk until it is combined. Add flour and salt to yeast mixture and combine until a dough forms. Knead dough about 10 minutes by hand, or about 4 minutes by mixer with a dough hook attachment. Place the dough in a bowl that has been lightly oiled and cover. Allow dough to rise at room temperature for about one hour - it should be doubled in size. Turn the risen dough out onto a floured table and knead 3 minutes or until all air is pressed out of dough. Divide dough into 3 equal pieces, and roll each one into a 12-15 inch long rope. Press the ends of the three ropes together, then braid the ropes, trying to keep the width of the loaf the same. Pinch the bottom ends together when you are done braiding it and place the loaf on a baking sheet that has been sprayed with nonstick cooking spray. Cover the loaf with a piece of plastic wrap that has also been sprayed with nonstick cooking spray and allow the dough to rise until again doubled in size, about an hour. While the dough is rising, preheat the oven to 400°F. Brush the loaf with a little beaten egg and place in the middle of the oven to bake for 20 - 30 minutes, or until the bread is a deep golden color. Transfer the loaf to a rack to cool completely before slicing.

Chocolate Bread

Serving Size: 10

1 3/4 cups all-purpose flour
1/4 cup unsweetened cocoa powder
1/2 tsp baking powder
1/2 tsp baking soda
1/2 tsp salt
2 large eggs
1/2 cup maltitol
1/4 cup brown sugar replacement
1/4 cup canola oil
3/4 cup lowfat sour cream

Preheat oven to 375°F and spray a 9X5X3 inch loaf pan with nonstick cooking spray, set aside. Sift flour, cocoa powder, baking powder and soda together, set aside. In another bowl, whip the eggs, maltitol and brown sugar replacement for about 3 minutes. While mixing, add the oil and sour cream. Add the liquid mixture to the dry ingredients and stir just until everything is combined. Pour the batter into the prepared pan and bake for about 50 minutes, or until a knife inserted in the center of the loaf comes out clean. Cool bread in pan for 10 minutes, then turn out onto a rack to finish cooling.

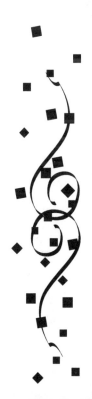

Chocolate Yeast Loaf

Serving Size: 10

1/4 cup warm water
1 tbsp maltitol
1/2 cup maltitol
1 package yeast
1 cup milk
2 tbsps butter, cut in pieces
4 cups bread flour
1 tsp salt
2/3 cup unsweetened cocoa powder
2 tsps instant coffee powder, not granules
2 large eggs
1 tsp vanilla extract
1/2 cup raisins, seedless

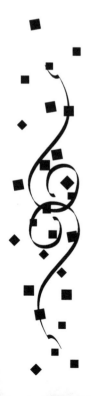

Mix the water and 1 tablespoon maltitol in mixing cup. Add
yeast and stir slightly. Set aside for 10 minutes until foamy.
Warm the milk and butter in a saucepan to about 110°F (butter
will not melt completely). In a large mixing bowl, combine 3-
3/4 cups flour, salt, cocoa, coffee and the remaining 1/2 cup
maltitol. Blend well. Beat eggs slightly and add the warm
milk, butter and vanilla; blend. Add this mixture along with
the yeast mixture to the flour. Stir in the raisins. Mix all with a
mixer with dough hook, or by hand with a wooden spoon.
Turn onto a lightly floured surface and knead for 5 to 6
minutes until smooth and elastic. Or continue mixing in the
mixer and knead only 2 minutes or so. Add more flour if
necessary. Grease a large bowl and place the dough into it,

continued on page 33

turning to grease all sides. Cover and let rise in a warm place until dough has doubled in size, about 2 hours. Knead the dough a few times, cover with plastic wrap and let rest for few minutes. Roll the dough into a large oval shape and roll up like a jelly roll, placing the seam side down. Roll from the narrow end to make it fit into the pan size you prefer. Use a loaf pan or a round casserole type pan. Butter a piece of plastic wrap and place loosely over the dough. Let rise again until doubled in size; about 1-1/2 hours. Preheat oven to 350°F and place bread near the center of the oven, not too high. Bake for 25 minutes, then cover loosely with foil and continue baking 30 to 40 minutes longer. Let cool for 10 minutes, then remove from pan and finish cooling on wire rack.

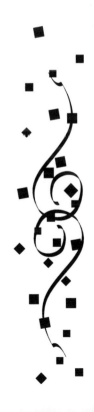

Easy Raisin Bread

Serving Size: 10

2 cups all-purpose flour
2 tsps baking powder
1/4 tsp salt
1/2 tsp baking soda
1 tsp cinnamon
1 egg
1 cup unsweetened applesauce
1/4 cup melted butter, cooled
1/2 cup maltitol
1 1/2 cups raisins, soaked in hot water

Preheat oven to 350°F and spray 9X5X3 inch loaf pan with nonstick cooking spray, set aside. Sift together first 5 ingredients, set aside. Combine egg, applesauce, melted butter and maltitol and mix until smooth. While mixing, add flour gradually until all ingredients are thoroughly combined. Remove raisins from hot water and squeeze out any excess water. Add raisins to batter, stir well, then pour into prepared loaf pan. Bake about 45 minutes, or until a knife inserted in the middle of the loaf comes out clean. Allow bread to cool before slicing.

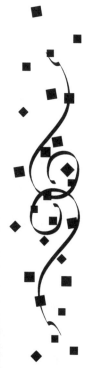

Quick Hints
Quick Muffin Topping
Sprinkle the tops of muffins with Grape-Nut cereal before baking for a quick, lowfat crunchy topping.

Honey Nut Bread

Serving Size: 20

1/2 cup margarine
1/2 cup light cream
3 tsps cinnamon
2 cups almonds, finely chopped
3 1/2 cups all-purpose flour
3 cups maltitol, honey flavored
2 tsps baking soda
1 1/2 tsps salt
1 tsp ground nutmeg
2 cups carrots, shredded
1 cup unsweetened applesauce
3/4 cup water
4 large eggs

Preheat oven to 350°F. Line two 9 x 5 x 3 inch loaf pans with aluminum foil. Then spray the foil with nonstick cooking spray, set aside. In a saucepan combine margarine, cream, and 2 teaspoons cinnamon. Bring to a boil, then reduce heat to medium-low and cook 1 minute. Stir in 1-1/2 cups finely chopped nuts. Cool mixture. Set aside. In a large mixing bowl, combine flour, maltitol, soda, salt, 1 teaspoon cinnamon and nutmeg. Stir in carrots and 1/2 cup finely chopped nuts. Combine applesauce, water and eggs; add to dry ingredients. Mix only until dry particles are moistened. Place 1 cup batter in each pan, then top with 1/2 cup nut mixture. Cover with another cup of batter then 1/2 cup nut mixture again. Finally top with remaining batter. Bake for 65-75 minutes. Center will crack and should feel dry to touch. Cool 15 minutes then remove from pan. Best if stored overnight before slicing.

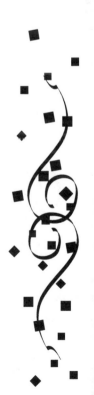

Irish Soda Bread

Serving Size: 8

3 cups all-purpose flour
1 tbsp maltitol
1 tsp salt
1 tsp baking soda
1 1/2 cups lowfat buttermilk

Sift together dry ingredients. Combine maltitol and buttermilk. Add liquid mixture to dry mixture and stir gently until everything is combined. Cover bowl and rest for 5 minutes. Preheat oven to 450°F. Remove the dough and knead for 1-2 minutes - just until it is smooth. Form the dough into a round loaf and place on a cookie sheet that has been sprayed with nonstick cooking spray. With a sharp knife, cut an X in the middle if the loaf, then let it rest for about 10 minutes. Bake the loaf for 45 minutes, or until it is a dark brown. Slide the bread onto a rack to cool.

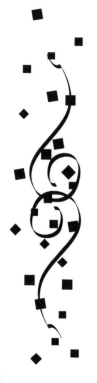

Lemon Bread

Serving Size: 10

3 tbsps butter, melted
1 cup maltitol
2 eggs
1 1/2 cups all-purpose flour
1/2 tsp salt
1/2 cup fresh lemon juice
2 tbsps lemon zest, grated

Preheat oven to 350°F and spray a 9X5X3 inch loaf pan with nonstick cooking spray. Stir maltitol into melted butter. Beat in eggs. Stir in flour and salt until just blended. Add lemon juice and lemon zest. Pour batter into loaf pan. Bake for 50 minutes. Remove from oven and cool ten minutes in pan. Turn out onto a rack to finish cooling.

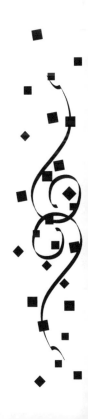

Mango Bread

Serving Size: 20

2 cups all-purpose flour
2 tsps baking soda
1/4 tsp salt
1 1/2 cups maltitol
3 large eggs, beaten
3/4 cup canola oil
2 cups mango, peeled and diced
1/2 cup chopped macadamia nuts
1 tbsp fresh lime juice

Preheat oven to 375°F and spray 2 8 1/2 X 4 1/2 X 3 inch loaf pans with nonstick cooking spray, set aside. Combine first 3 ingredients and make a well in the center of the mixture. Combine remaining ingredients and add to flour mixture. Stir until all ingredients are thoroughly combined. Pour into the two prepared pans and bake for 1 hour or until a knife inserted in the center comes out clean. Cool in pans 10 minutes before removing to a wire rack to cool completely.

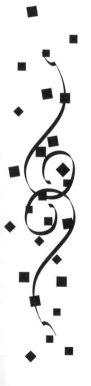

Pumpkin Quick Bread

Serving Size: 10

1 1/2 cups all-purpose flour
1/2 cup rolled oats, ground in blender
2 tsps baking powder
2 tsps baking soda
2 tsps cinnamon
2 tsps nutmeg
1/4 tsp allspice
1 tsp ground ginger
3/4 cup maltitol, maple flavored
1/4 cup canola oil
2 egg whites
1 whole egg
2 tbsps lemon juice
1 tbsp grated orange zest
1 cup canned pumpkin puree

Preheat oven to 350°F and spray a 9X5X3 inch loaf pan with nonstick cooking spray, set aside. In a large mixing bowl, combine flour, oats, baking powder, baking soda, cinnamon, nutmeg, allspice and ginger. In a separate bowl combine maltitol, oil, egg whites, egg, lemon juice, orange peel, and pumpkin. Combine contents of both bowls, mixing very lightly. Pour into prepared loaf pan and bake for 50 to 60 minutes. Let cool before slicing.

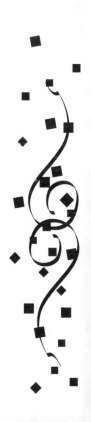

Sticky Nut Buns

Serving Size: 24

6 cups all-purpose flour
1/3 cup maltitol, honey flavored
1 tsp salt
1/2 tsp lemon rind, grated
2 packages dry yeast
1 cup butter
2 large eggs
Filling:
1/3 cup maltitol, honey flavored
1 cup pecans, chopped
2 egg yolks
1 tsp lemon peel, grated

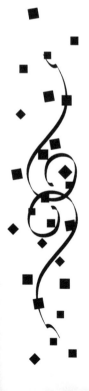

Place 1-1/2 cups flour in a large bowl. Add maltitol, salt, lemon peel and yeast. Soften butter and add to flour mixture. Add 1-1/3 cups very warm (120°-130°F) water to the flour mixture and beat 2 minutes at medium speed; scrape bowl occasionally. Add eggs and 1/2 cup flour; beat at high speed for 2 minutes, scraping bowl occasionally. Stir in more flour to make a soft dough. Cover and let rest for 20 minutes. Turn dough out onto well-floured surface; divide into 3 parts. Roll each piece to an 8-inch square. Cut each square into eight 1-inch strips. Twist each strip and coil in a circle, sealing ends underneath. Place on greased cookie sheet. Make a wide indentation in center of each roll, pressing to the bottom. To make filling, combine 1/3 cup maltitol and 1 cup finely chopped pecans in a saucepan. Bring to a boil and simmer over low heat for 3 minutes. Gradually stir in beaten egg yolks and cook, stirring, until slightly thickened. Stir in lemon peel then cool. Spoon filling into indentations, using 1 teaspoon for each roll. Repeat with each piece of dough. Cover loosely and let rise in warm place until doubled in bulk. Bake in preheated 375°F oven for 15-20 minutes or until done.

Zucchini Bread

Serving Size: 20

3 eggs
3/4 cup canola oil
1/4 cup unsweetened applesauce
1 1/2 cups maltitol
2 cups zucchini unpeeled, grated
2 tsps vanilla extract
3 cups all-purpose flour
1 tsp salt
1 tsp baking soda
1 tbsp cinnamon
1/2 tsp baking powder

Preheat oven to 325°F and spray two 9X5X3 inch loaf pans
with nonstick cooking spray, set aside. Beat eggs until light
and foamy, then add in oil, applesauce, maltitol, zucchini and
vanilla, mixing lightly but well. Sift flour, salt, soda,
cinnamon, and baking powder and mix until well blended.
Divide batter between the 2 pans and bake for an hour or until
a knife inserted in the center comes out clean. Remove loaves
from pans and cool on a rack. This bread also freezes
beautifully.
Notes: To reduce the fat in this bread a little, use 1/2
    cup applesauce and 1/2 cup canola oil. The bread
    turns out the same, but dries out a little faster.

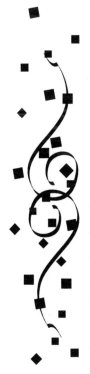

Blueberry Muffins

Serving Size: 24

1/4 cup vegetable shortening
2 large eggs
2 cups all-purpose flour
2 1/2 tsp double-acting baking powder
2 tsp maltitol
3/4 cup skim milk
1 cup blueberries

Preheat oven to 375°F and lightly spray small muffin tin with nonstick cooking spray. Cream shortening in mixing bowl. Add eggs and mix well. Sift flour and baking powder together. Add flour mixture, maltitol syrup and milk alternately to shortening. Stir well after each addition. Batter will be stiff. Fold in blueberries. Fill each muffin cup 1/2 full of batter. Bake for about 20 minutes or until browned.

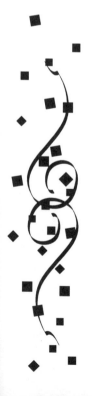

Buttermilk Biscuits

Serving Size: 12

2 1/2 cups all-purpose flour
2 1/2 tsp baking powder
1/2 tsp baking soda
1/4 tsp salt
6 tbsp margarine, cold
1 cup lowfat buttermilk

Preheat oven to 500°F and lightly spray a baking sheet with nonstick cooking spray, set aside. Sift together dry ingredients, then cut in margarine with a pastry blender until the mixture looks like coarse cornmeal. Stir in the buttermilk with a fork - if the dough is really moist, add as little flour as possible to make it easy to handle. Place the dough on a floured table and knead it about 10 times, then pat the dough 1/2 inch thick. Cut out biscuits and place them on prepared pan. Any scraps that are left over can be kneaded together and patted out again. Bake biscuits 10-12 minutes, or until they are golden. Serve immediately.

Notes: A great way to make biscuits extra tasty is to take about 1/2-3/4 cup of vegetables and chop them finely in a food processor, then add them to the biscuit mixture with the buttermilk. A combination of broccoli, carrots, bell peppers and squash is delicious.

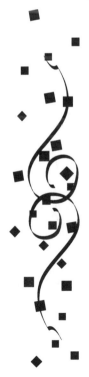

Carrot Muffins

Serving Size: 12

1/3 cup chopped pecans
1/3 cup water
2 1/2 cups all-purpose flour
2 teaspoons cinnamon
2 teaspoons baking soda
2 cups grated carrots
1 cup crushed pineapple, drained
1/4 cup canola oil
1/2 cup maltitol
1/2 cup raisins, soaked in hot water
3 egg whites

Preheat oven to 350°F and spray a muffin tin with nonstick cooking spray, set aside. Place pecans and the water in a blender and puree, then strain milk into a bowl. Set aside. In a large bowl sift together flour, cinnamon, and baking soda. In a separate bowl combine pecan milk, carrots, pineapple, canola oil, maltitol, and raisins. In a smaller bowl beat egg whites until stiff peaks form. Mix dry and wet ingredients, stirring briefly to combine. Fold in egg whites. Spoon batter into muffin tin and bake for 35 minutes. Let cool, then remove from muffin tin.

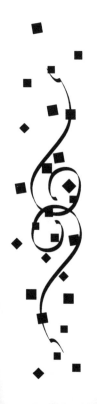

Carrot-Ginger Muffins

Serving Size: 12

2 cups all-purpose flour
1 tbsp baking powder
1 tsp baking soda
1/2 tsp nutmeg
1/2 tsp cinnamon
2 tsp grated gingerroot
1/2 cup lowfat buttermilk
1/4 cup canola oil
1/2 cup maltitol, maple flavored
3 eggs
2 cups grated carrot

Preheat oven to 400°F and spray a muffin tin with nonstick cooking spray. In a large bowl combine flour, baking powder, baking soda, nutmeg, and cinnamon. In a separate bowl combine gingerroot, buttermilk, canola oil, maltitol syrup, and eggs. Stir together contents of both bowls, then stir in carrots. Spoon into muffin tins, filling about three quarters full, and bake for 15 to 18 minutes. Remove from pan and serve warm.

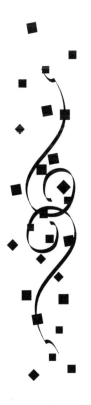

Chocolate Muffins

Serving Size: 12

4 1/2 ounces unsweetened chocolate squares
1/3 cup canola oil
3/4 cup lowfat sour cream
2/3 cup brown sugar replacement
1/2 cup maltitol
1 egg
2 tsp vanilla extract
1 1/2 cups all-purpose flour
1 tsp baking soda
1/4 tsp salt
1/2 cup raisins, soaked in hot water

Preheat oven to 400°F and spray muffin tin with nonstick cooking spray, set aside. Mix chocolate and canola oil together; melt over simmering water in double boiler. Allow to cool to lukewarm. Mix sour cream, brown sugar replacement, maltitol syrup, egg and vanilla. Blend with melted chocolate. Blend flour, soda and salt; add the chocolate mixture and blend very well. Add the raisins (you can omit them, if desired). Pour batter into muffin tins. Bake for about 20 minutes. Remove from muffin tins and allow to cool on wire racks.

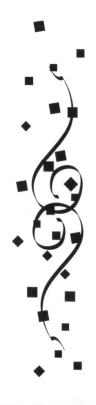

Cran-Apple Muffins

Serving Size: 18

2 cups peeled apples, shredded
1 1/3 cups maltitol
1 cup cranberries, chopped
1 cup carrots, shredded
2 1/2 cups all-purpose flour
1 tbsp double-acting baking powder
2 tsp baking soda
1/2 tsp salt
2 tsp ground cinnamon
2 eggs, beaten
1/2 cup vegetable oil

In a large mixing bowl, combine apples and maltitol syrup.
Gently fold in chopped cranberries and carrots. Combine dry
ingredients; add to mixing bowl. Mix well to moisten dry
ingredients. Combine eggs and oil; stir into apple mixture. Fill
18 greased muffin tins 2/3 full. Bake at 375°F for 20-25
minutes. Cool 5 minutes before removing from pans.

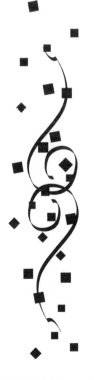

Farina Muffins

Serving Size: 10

1 egg, beaten
4 tablespoons shortening, liquid
3/4 cup milk
3/4 cup Malt-o-Meal®
1 1/4 cups flour
1/2 cup maltitol
3 teaspoons baking powder

Mix all ingredients just until moistened; DO NOT overmix.
Fill muffin cups 3/4 full. Bake in preheated 400-degree oven
for 20 minutes.

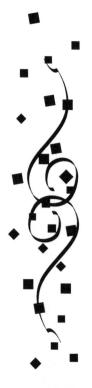

Fat Free Oatmeal-Raisin Muffins

Serving Size: 24

2 cups all-purpose flour
1/2 cup oatmeal
1/2 cup maltitol
1 tbsp double-acting baking powder
1/2 tsp salt
1 1/2 tsp cinnamon
1 cup raisins, soaked in hot water
4 egg whites
1 1/3 cups skim milk
1/4 cup unsweetened applesauce

Preheat oven to 350°F, spray two 12-cup muffin pans with nonstick cooking spray. Fit the steel knife blade into the work bowl of a food processor. Combine all ingredients in the bowl. Process until batter is smooth, 10-15 seconds, stopping once to scrape down sides of bowl with rubber spatula. Raisins should be in large pieces. Spoon batter into prepared muffin cups. Bake until a wooden pick inserted in center of muffin comes out clean, about 25 minutes.

Variation: Pour batter into a greased 9X5 loaf pan. Bake until a wooden pick inserted in center comes out clean, about 1 hour.

Notes: If all the muffins are not to be eaten the day they are baked, freeze the remaining muffins because they dry out faster than muffins with fat in them.

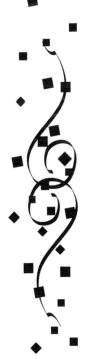

Gingerbread Muffins

Serving Size: 12

1 cup butter
1/2 cup brown sugar replacement
4 eggs
2 1/2 cups all-purpose flour
1 cup maltitol
2 tsp cinnamon
2 tsp baking soda
1 cup lowfat buttermilk
2 tsp ground ginger
2 cups whole-wheat flour

Preheat oven to 350°F and spray muffin tin with nonstick cooking spray. Cream butter and brown sugar replacement. Add eggs, one at a time, beating after each. Add maltitol syrup. Sift flours, baking soda. and spices. Add alternately with buttermilk. Fill muffin pans 2/3 full and bake 15 minutes or until muffins spring back when you press on them lightly. Cool on a wire rack or enjoy warm.

Notes: These muffins do not have the rich molasses flavor that most gingerbread does, however, if you can ingest small amounts of sugar, try replacing some of the maltitol syrup with a little molasses.

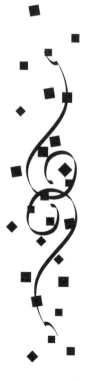

Low Fat Oat Bran Muffins

Serving Size: 12

2 cups oat bran
2 cups whole wheat pastry flour
3/4 cup raisins, soaked in hot water
1 1/2 tsp baking soda
2/3 cup maltitol, honey flavored
2 cups lowfat buttermilk

Preheat oven to 350°F and spray a muffin tin with nonstick cooking spray. In a large bowl, combine bran, flour, raisins, and baking soda. Stir together maltitol syrup and buttermilk, then pour over bran mixture. Let stand for 20 minutes. Fill muffin cups two thirds full of batter and bake until muffins spring back slightly when pressed in the center, about 30 minutes. Remove from pan and serve warm.

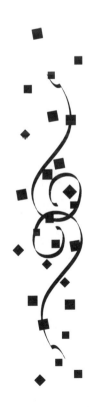

Pineapple Muffins

Serving Size: 12

1 cup crushed pineapple
3/4 cup skim milk
1 large egg, beaten
2 cups all-purpose flour
1 tbsp double-acting baking powder
1/4 tsp salt
1/4 tsp ground nutmeg, optional
1/4 cup maltitol
1/4 cup canola oil

Preheat oven to 400°F and lightly spray muffin tin with
nonstick cooking spray, set aside. Drain pineapple, reserving
juice. Place juice into a measuring cup, adding milk to equal
one cup. Combine with the beaten egg. Sift together in large
bowl flour, baking powder and salt. Blend milk mixture into
dry ingredients, alternating with canola oil mixed with
maltitol syrup. Mix until just blended. Stir in drained
pineapple. Pour into muffin tins. Bake for 18-22 minutes, or
until golden brown.

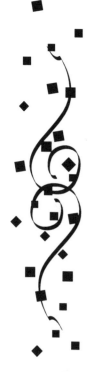

Sweet Potato Muffins

Serving Size: 12

1/2 cup butter, softened
1 cup maltitol
1/2 cup brown sugar replacement
1 cup sweet potato puree
1 egg
1 3/4 cups flour
1/4 teaspoon salt
1/2 teaspoon ground nutmeg
1/2 teaspoon ground ginger
1 teaspoon baking soda
2 teaspoons ground cinnamon
1/8 teaspoon ground cloves
1/3 cup water

Preheat oven to 375°F and spray a muffin tin with nonstick cooking spray. Cream the butter and maltitol syrup together until light and fluffy. Mix in the sweet potato and egg. Sift together flour, salt, nutmeg, ginger, baking soda, cinnamon, and cloves. Stir half the dry ingredients into creamed mixture; stir in water, then add the remaining dry ingredients. Fill muffin cups two thirds full of batter; bake 18 to 20 minutes, or until dry on top and a skewer inserted in center comes out clean.

Serving Ideas: Best when served warm.

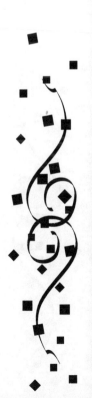

Wheat Germ Muffins

Serving Size: 12

1 1/2 cups all-purpose flour
2 tsp baking powder
1 tsp salt
1 cup wheat germ
3/4 cup milk
1/4 cup butter
1 large egg
1/2 cup maltitol

Preheat oven to 400°F and lightly spray 12 muffin tins with
nonstick cooking spray, set aside. In a mixing bowl, combine
flour, baking powder and salt. Melt butter and beat the egg
well and combine them both with the maltitol syrup. Add to
the flour mixture along with rest of ingredients. Stir just
enough to moisten ingredients, batter will be lumpy. Fill each
muffin cup 2/3 full and sprinkle a little additional wheat
germ on top, if desired. Bake for 15 minutes or until browned
on top.

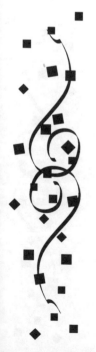

cakes

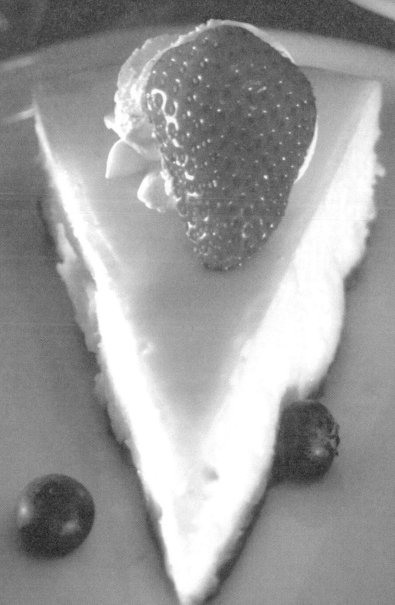

Chocolate Cheesecake

Serving Size: 12

1 recipe chocolate tart dough *(recipe on page 261)*
1 envelope unflavored gelatin
1/4 cup cold water
16 ounces cream cheese, softened
5 1/4 tsps Equal® sweetener
1/3 cup unsweetened cocoa powder, sifted
1 tsp vanilla extract
1 cup heavy cream

Roll out tart crust to 1/4 inch thick and line the bottom only of a 9 or 10 inch springform pan with it. Bake at 325 for 20 minutes. Set aside. Sprinkle gelatin over cold water in a small saucepan and let sit for 5 minutes. Place saucepan over low heat and stir until gelatin has dissolved, but do not boil the mixture. Set aside. Combine cream cheese, Equal, cocoa and vanilla and mix until well blended. Gradually add gelatin mixture to cream cheese, mixing until all ingredients are thoroughly combined. Place mixture, covered, in refrigerator until it is slightly thickened, about one hour. Whip heavy cream until soft peaks form, then gently fold it into cream cheese mixture. Pour it over prepared crust and chill until firm, preferably overnight.

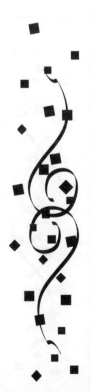

Plain Cheesecake

Serving Size: 8

1 recipe sweet tart dough *(recipe on page 265)*
1 envelope unflavored gelatin
1/4 cup cold water
8 ounces cream cheese, softened
3 1/2 tsps Equal® sweetener
1/2 cup skim milk
1 tsp grated lemon rind, yellow part only
1/4 cup fresh lemon juice
1 cup heavy cream

Line the bottom of a 9 or 10 inch springform pan with 1/4 inch thick piece of tart dough and bake 20 minutes at 325°F. Set aside. Sprinkle gelatin over cold water and let sit for 5 minutes. Place saucepan over low heat and stir until gelatin is dissolved, but do not boil. Set aside. Combine cream cheese and Equal and mix until very creamy. Gradually add milk, lemon zest and juice, then gelatin mixture, mixing until well blended. Place mixture, covered, in refrigerator until slightly thickened, about one hour. Whip heavy cream until soft peaks form, then gently fold it into the cream cheese mixture. Pour over prepared crust and chill until firm, preferably overnight. Garnish with berries, if desired.

Notes: The best way to cut a cheesecake is to take a knife and run it under hot water so it is slightly warmed and then cut the piece. Repeat for each slice cut and the cheesecake will not stick to the knife.

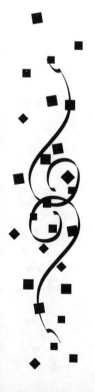

Praline Cheesecake

Serving Size: 12

1 recipe Nutty Tart Crust made with pecans *(recipe on*
    page 262)
2 pounds cream cheese
1/2 cup maltitol
1/2 cup brown sugar replacement
4 eggs
2 tbsps bourbon
1 cup chopped pecans, toasted

Preheat oven to 325°F. Roll out tart dough so that it covers the
bottom only of a 9-10 inch springform pan a little less than
1/4 inch thick. Bake the crust for 20 minutes. Turn oven down
to 325°F. Place cream cheese in a bowl and mix until it is soft,
then gradually add the maltitol and brown sugar replacement.
Scrape bowl. Add eggs, one at a time, scraping the bowl
between each addition. Add bourbon, then scrape the bowl
again. Finally add pecans and stir just until mixed. Pour
cheesecake mixture into the prepared pan and place the pan in
a larger pan. Place 1 inch of warm water in the larger pan and
place it in the oven. Bake the cake for about 1 hour or until it
is set and lightly browned on the edges. Remove the
springform pan from the water bath and let the cake cool
completely before serving.

Notes: Because this cheesecake is baked in a water bath, it is
        important that your springform pan is tight and no
        water leaks in. Test this ahead of time and if it does
        leak, try wrapping the bottom of the pan in a couple
        layers of foil.

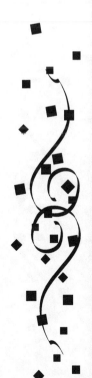

Raspberry Cheesecake

Serving Size: 12

1 recipe chocolate tart dough *(recipe on page 261)*
1 1/2 pounds cream cheese
3/4 cup maltitol
2 tbsps all-purpose flour
1 tsp vanilla
2 eggs
1 egg yolk
1/2 cup raspberry liqueur
 fresh raspberries for garnish, optional

Roll out tart dough and place on the bottom and 1 inch up the
sides of the springform pan. Mix cream cheese until it is soft
then gradually add maltitol to it while mixing. Add flour and
vanilla and mix well. Scrape down sides of bowl. Add egg
and egg yolk all at once, mix well, then scrape down sides
and bottom. Mix in raspberry liqueur. Pour filling into
prepared pan and place in a 375°F oven for 35-40 minutes or
until center is almost set. Cool cheesecake in pan.

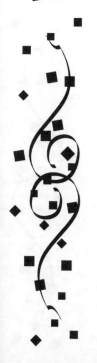

Three Cheese Cheese Cake

Serving Size: 10

1 recipe sweet tart dough *(recipe on page 265)*
1 pound cottage cheese, creamed
1 pound cream cheese, softened
1 1/2 cups maltitol
4 eggs
1 tsp vanilla extract
3 tbsps all-purpose flour
3 tbsps cornstarch
1/4 cup butter, melted
1 pint sour cream

Preheat oven to 325°F and line the bottom of the springform pan with tart dough. Cream cottage cheese and cream cheese. Gradually add maltitol, beating well. Add eggs one at a time, beating well between each. Stir in vanilla. Sift over all flour and cornstarch, blend in. Add melted butter and mix until smooth. Blend in sour cream. Pour into spring form pan. Bake for one hour. Turn off oven and let cake remain in the oven for 2 more hours. Chill.

Notes: To cream cottage cheese, place it in a blender and blend until smooth.

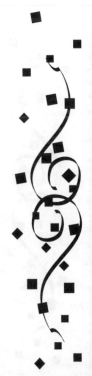

Almond Meringue Torte

Serving Size: 8

1/4 cup maltitol
1/2 cup all-purpose flour
1/2 tsp cream of tartar
1/4 tsp double-acting baking soda
1/4 cup butter
1 egg yolk, lightly beaten
2 egg whites
1/4 cup maltitol
1/4 cup ground almonds
1/3 cup apricot all-fruit preserves

Preheat oven to 350°F and spray a 8 inch square pan with nonstick cooking spray. Sift together dry ingredients. Cut butter into dry ingredients. Stir in egg yolk. Pat into pan. Bake for 15 minutes. Increase oven temperature to 450°F. While cake bakes, beat egg white until stiff, and beat in maltitol. Gently fold in ground almonds. When cake is set and light golden brown, remove from oven, spread with jam and then almond meringue mixture. Brown at 450°F for 5-10 minutes.

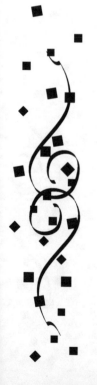

Banana Nut Cake

Serving Size: 10

1 recipe nut cake *(recipe on page 72)*
1 recipe banana buttercream *(recipe on page 267)*
banana chips, optional
nuts, optional

Place one layer of cake on a cake plate and spread the top
with frosting. Place the other layer on top and spread it with
frosting. Spread frosting on the sides of the cake as smoothly
as possible. Garnish the cake with banana chips around the
top edge and nuts pressed against the sides, if desired.

Black and White Cake

Serving Size: 10

1 recipe chocolate cake, cooked & cooled
    (recipe on page 66)
1 recipe vanilla buttercream *(recipe on page 272)*
grated sugar free fudge, optional

Place a cake layer on a cake plate and spread the top with
frosting. Place the other layer on top and spread it with
frosting. Spread the frosting all around the cake and garnish
with sprinkles of grated fudge, if desired.

Notes: The flavor of vanilla compliments and brings out the
        most flavor in chocolate.

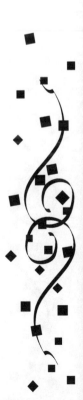

Carrot Cake

Serving Size: 10

2 cups all-purpose flour
1 tsp baking powder
1 tsp baking soda
1 tsp cinnamon
1/4 tsp allspice
1 3/4 cups maltitol
3 cups shredded carrots
1/4 cup unsweetened applesauce
1/2 cup canola oil
4 eggs beaten
1 tsp vanilla extract
1 cup chopped pecans, optional

Preheat oven to 350°F and spray two 9 inch round cake pans with nonstick cooking spray and set aside. Sift first five ingredients together and set aside. Combine remaining ingredients, except pecans, then add flour mixture to it, and mix until well combined. Stir in pecans, then pour cake into prepared pans. Bake 30-35 minutes, or until a toothpick inserted in the center of the cake comes out clean. Allow cakes to cool 10 minutes in the pan before turning out onto a rack to cool completely before icing.

Notes: This cake is best when iced with the traditional cream cheese icing.

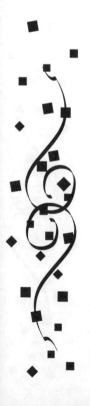

Chocolate and Grand Marnier Cake

Serving Size: 10

1 recipe chocolate cake, cooked & cooled
   (recipe on page 66)
1/2 cup Grand Marnier
1 recipe orange buttercream *(recipe on page 272)*
1 orange sliced

Place chocolate cake on a cake platter and soak the layer with 1/4 cup Grand Marnier. Spread the top with buttercream and put the other layer on top. Soak the second layer with the remaining Grand Marnier and cover it in buttercream. Ice the sides of the cake with the frosting. Garnish the cake with orange slices.

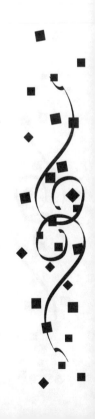

Chocolate Cake

Serving Size: 10

4 ounces unsweetened chocolate squares
1/4 cup coffee
1 1/2 cups maltitol
1/2 cup butter, softened
1 tsp vanilla extract
3 eggs
2 cups cake flour sifted
1 tsp baking soda
1/4 tsp salt
2/3 cup skim milk

Preheat oven to 350°F. Spray 2 9-inch round pans with nonstick cooking spray and set aside. Combine chocolate, coffee, and 1/2 cup maltitol in a small pan and stir over low heat until chocolate is melted and mixture is smooth. Set aside to cool. In a large bowl, whip butter with mixer on high until it is white and fluffy, then gradually mix in the remaining maltitol. Add vanilla, then eggs, one at a time, beating thoroughly after each addition. Sift the cake flour, baking soda and salt together, and add it to the batter alternately with the milk until all are blended. Beat in the chocolate mixture until it is completely mixed in. Pour batter into the two pans and bake on middle rack for 35-40 minutes, or until a toothpick comes out clean. Cool cakes in the pans 10 minutes before turning out on a rack to cool. Cool cakes completely before icing.

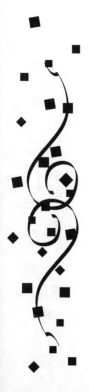

Chocolate Lovers Cake

Serving Size: 10

1 recipe chocolate cake, cooked & cooled
    (recipe on page 66)
1 recipe ganache, slightly beaten *(recipe on page 270)*
 grated sugar free fudge, optional

Ice cake layers with ganache on top of each layer and on all
the sides. Sprinkle grated fudge all over the cake.

Chocolate Raspberry Torte

Serving Size: 10

1 recipe chocolate cake, cooked & cooled
    (recipe on page 66)
10 1/2 ounces all-fruit raspberry preserves, no sugar
    added
1 recipe ganache, warmed *(recipe on page 270)*
3 tbsps raspberry liqueur

Split the cake layers in half so that you have four equal layers.
Spread the raspberry preserves evenly between three layers,
place them on top of each other, with the top layer not having
any preserves on it. Heat the ganache so that it is pourable
and stir in the raspberry liqueur. Place the cake on a rack and
pour the ganache over the cake. Let the cake sit until the
ganache has hardened some.

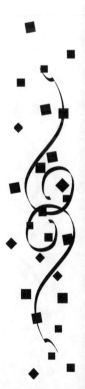

Classic Carrot Cake

Serving Size: 10

1 recipe carrot cake, cooked & cooled *(recipe on page 64)*
1 recipe cream cheese frosting *(recipe on page 269)*
 pecans for garnish, optional

Place carrot cake layer on a cake plate and spread top with
frosting. Place next layer on top and spread with icing.
Smooth icing around sides of cake. Press chopped pecans into
the sides of the cake, if desired.

Dinner Mint Cake

Serving Size: 10

1 recipe chocolate cake, cooked & cooled
     (recipe on page 66)
1 recipe creme de menthe buttercream
     (recipe on page 270)
 grated sugar free fudge, optional

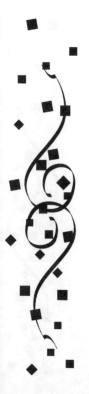

Place one cake layer on a cake plate and spread with frosting.
Put the other layer on top and spread with frosting. Ice the
sides of the cake so that they are as smooth as possible.
Sprinkle grated fudge over the cake.

Notes: If desired, the cake can be soaked with 1/4 cup of
        creme de menthe on each layer.

German Chocolate Cake

Serving Size: 10

1 recipe chocolate cake, cooked & cooled
    (recipe on page 66)
1 recipe coconut and pecan frosting, cooled
    (recipe on page 268)
 pecan halves for garnish, optional

Place one cake layer on a cake plate and spread it with half of the frosting. Place the other layer on top and spread the remaining frosting on top. Garnish with additional pecan halves around the edges, if desired.

Italian Creme Cake

Serving Size: 10

1 recipe vanilla cake *(recipe on page 77)*
1 recipe cream cheese frosting *(recipe on page 269)*
2 cups unsweetened coconut

Ice cake with cream cheese frosting and press shredded coconut all over the sides and top of cake, and in between the layers.

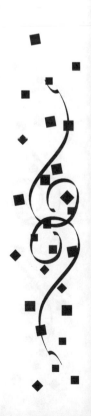

Lemon Pecan Cake

Serving Size: 10

1 recipe nut cake made with pecans *(recipe on page 72)*
1 recipe lemon buttercream *(recipe on page 271)*
 chopped pecans, optional

Place a cake layer on a cake plate and spread with frosting.
Place the other layer on top and repeat. Spread the sides of the
cake with frosting and press chopped pecans into the sides.

Lemony Cake

Serving Size: 10

1 recipe vanilla cake *(recipe on page 77)*
1 recipe lemon buttercream *(recipe on page 271)*
 grated sugar free white fudge

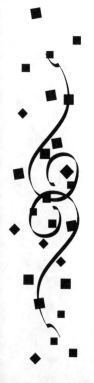

Place one layer of cake on a cake platter and spread with
frosting. Place the other layer on top and spread with frosting.
Spread frosting all over the sides as smooth as possible.
Sprinkle the cake with the grated fudge, if desired.

Light Vanilla Cake

Serving Size: 10

1 recipe vanilla cake, cooked & cooled
   (recipe on page 77)
1 recipe 7 Minute Frosting *(recipe on page 266)*
 grated sugar free white fudge, optional

Place one layer of cake on a cake platter and spread with frosting. Place the other layer on top and spread with frosting. Spread frosting all over the sides as smooth as possible. Press grated fudge into the sides of the cake, if desired.

Mocha Cake

Serving Size: 10

1 recipe chocolate cake, cooked & cooled
   (recipe on page 66)
1 recipe coffee buttercream *(recipe on page 269)*
1/2 cup coffee liqueur
 grated sugar free fudge, optional

Soak both layers of cake with 1/4 cup of liqueur each. Ice cake on top of both layers and around the edges. Sprinkle grated fudge all over cake.

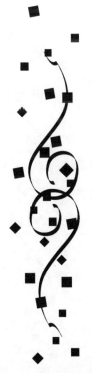

Nut Cake

Serving Size: 10

12 tbsps unsalted butter, softened
1 cup maltitol
1/2 cup brown sugar replacement
3 large eggs
2 cups all-purpose flour
1 cup nuts, ground very fine
1 tsp baking powder
1 tsp baking soda
1 cup lowfat buttermilk

Preheat oven to 350°F and spray two 9 inch round pans with nonstick cooking spray, set aside. In a large mixing bowl, whip the butter until it is very fluffy and white. Gradually add the maltitol and brown sugar replacement. Add the eggs, one at a time, and beat well after each addition. Sift together flour, baking powder and soda, then stir in nuts to the flour mixture. Add 1/3 of the four mixture to the butter mixture, then add 1/3 of the buttermilk. Repeat until all ingredients are used up. Pour the batter into the prepared pans and bake the cakes for 25-30 minutes, or until a toothpick inserted in the center comes out clean. Cool the cakes in the pans for 10 minutes before turning out onto a rack to cool completely.

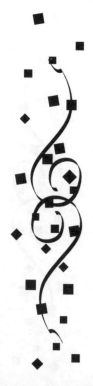

Peppermint Cake

Serving Size: 10

1 recipe vanilla cake *(recipe on page 77)*
1 recipe creme de menthe buttercream
  (recipe on page 270)
 crushed sugar free peppermints, optional

Place one layer of cake on a cake platter and spread with
frosting. Place the other layer on top and spread with frosting.
Spread frosting all over the sides as smooth as possible.
Sprinkle the cake with the crushed peppermints, if desired.

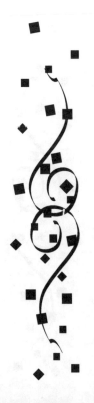

Spice Cake

Serving Size: 10

1/2 cup butter, softened
1 1/2 cups maltitol
1 tsp vanilla extract
3 eggs
1 cup lowfat buttermilk
2 cups all-purpose flour
1 tsp baking soda
1 1/2 tsps cinnamon
1/4 tsp ground nutmeg
1/4 tsp ground cloves
1/4 tsp allspice
1/4 tsp ground ginger

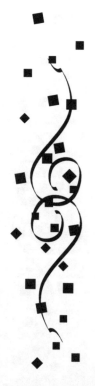

Preheat oven to 350°F and spray two 9 inch round pans with nonstick cooking spray, set aside. In one bowl, whip butter until fluffy and white, then slowly add maltitol while still mixing. Add vanilla, then eggs, one at a time, beating well after each addition. Mix in buttermilk and set aside. Sift remaining ingredients together in another bowl, then add them to the liquid mixture a little at a time. Pour batter into pans and bake 20-25 minutes or until a toothpick inserted in the center of the cake comes out clean. Cool in pan 10 minutes before turning it out onto a rack to cool completely.

Spice Cake with Cream Cheese Frosting

Serving Size: 10

1 recipe spice cake, cooked & cooled *(recipe on page 74)*
1 recipe cream cheese frosting *(recipe on page 269)*
 cinnamon, optional

Place one layer of cake on a cake platter and spread with
frosting. Place the other layer on top and spread with frosting.
Spread frosting all over the sides as smooth as possible. To
make a pretty design on top of the cake, place a paper doily
on top of it and sprinkle cinnamon over it. Carefully remove
the doily.

Spice Cake with Vanilla Icing

Serving Size: 10

1 recipe spice cake, cooked & cooled *(recipe on page 74)*
1 recipe 7 Minute Frosting *(recipe on page 266)*
 chopped nuts, optional

Place one layer of cake on a cake platter and spread with
frosting. Place the other layer on top and spread with frosting.
Spread frosting all over the sides as smooth as possible.
Sprinkle the cake with chopped nuts, if desired.

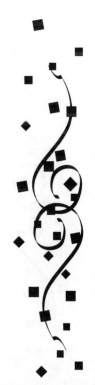

Strawberry Cake

Serving Size: 10

1 recipe vanilla cake, cooked & cooled
    (recipe on page 77)
1 recipe vanilla buttercream *(recipe on page 272)*
1/2 recipe pastry cream
1 pint strawberries, washed and sliced

Place one layer of cake on a cake platter and spread with
pastry cream. Top the pastry cream with a single layer of
strawberry slices. Place the other layer on top and spread with
frosting. Spread frosting all over the sides as smooth as
possible. Arrange strawberries on top of cake so that they
overlap each other just a little.

Vanilla Almond Cake

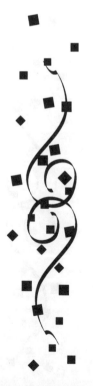

Serving Size: 10

1 recipe nut cake made with almonds *(recipe on page 72)*
1 recipe vanilla buttercream *(recipe on page 272)*
slivered almonds, optional
grated sugar free white fudge, optional

Place one layer of cake on a cake platter and spread with
frosting. Place the other layer on top and spread with frosting.
Spread frosting all over the sides as smooth as possible. Press
slivered almonds into the sides of the cake and top with
grated white fudge, if desired.

Vanilla Cake

Serving Size: 10

3 cups cake flour, sifted
1 tbsp baking powder
1/2 tsp salt
1/2 cup shortening
1 1/2 cups maltitol
1 tsp vanilla extract
1 cup skim milk
1/2 cup egg whites at room temperature

Preheat oven to 350°F and spray two 9 inch pans with nonstick cooking spray and set them aside. Sift together cake flour, baking powder and salt and set aside. Whip shortening five minutes, then slowly add maltitol and vanilla while whipping. Add sifted flour mixture and milk alternately to the butter mixture in small amounts, beating well after each addition. Wash beater of mixer until no oils are left on them, then beat the egg whites in a separate bowl until stiff peaks form, but not until they are dry. Carefully fold egg whites into the batter then pour into prepared pans. Bake 30-35 minutes, or until a toothpick inserted in the middle of the cake comes out clean. Allow cakes to cool in pans 10 minutes before turning them out onto racks to cool completely before icing.

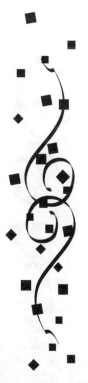

Apple Cake

Serving Size: 12

3 eggs
1/4 cup canola oil
1/2 cup unsweetened applesauce
2 tsps vanilla extract
1 1/2 cups maltitol
2 1/4 cups flour
1 1/2 cups maltitol
1 1/2 tsps ground cinnamon
1/4 tsp ground nutmeg
3/4 tsp baking soda
3/4 tsp baking powder
1/2 tsp salt
3 cups peeled apples, cored & diced
1 1/2 cups pecans, chopped

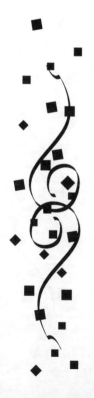

Preheat oven to 375°F and spray a 13X9X2 inch baking pan
with nonstick cooking spray. In large bowl of electric mixer,
beat eggs, oil, applesauce, vanilla and maltitol until well
combined. Combine flour, cinnamon, nutmeg, baking soda,
baking powder, and salt, stirring to combine thoroughly. Add
to egg mixture and stir to blend. Stir in apples and nuts.
Spoon batter into baking pan. Bake 30 to 40 minutes, or until a
skewer inserted in center comes out clean. Cool 30 minutes in
pan on rack before cutting.

Notes: Great when served warm with creme anglaise.

Apple Walnut Cake

Serving Size: 12

2 cups maltitol
1/2 cup margarine
2 large eggs
2 tsps vanilla extract
2 tsps baking soda
1 tsp salt
2 cups all-purpose flour
1 tsp ground cinnamon
4 cups Golden delicious apples sliced thin
1 cup black walnuts chopped

Cream margarine and maltitol in mixing bowl. Add beaten eggs and vanilla extract and whisk to blend well. Combine baking soda, salt, flour and cinnamon; add to egg mixture and beat until thoroughly mixed. Add peeled and thinly sliced apples along with the chopped walnuts to batter. Blend only enough to spread apples and nuts throughout batter. Spray a 13x9x2-inch pan with nonstick cooking spray. Pour in the batter and bake in a preheated 325°F oven for 1 hour.

Serving Ideas: Serve warm or cold with a dollop of whipped cream.

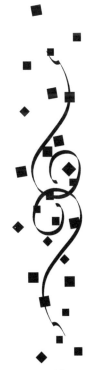

Applesauce Prune Cake

Serving Size: 12

1/2 cup margarine
1 cup maltitol
1 egg
1 2/3 cups all-purpose flour
1 tsp baking powder
1 tsp baking soda
2 tsps ground cinnamon
3/4 tsp allspice
1 cup dried prunes, chopped
1/2 cup chopped pecans
1 cup unsweetened applesauce

Preheat oven to 350°F and spray a 9 cup bundt pan with nonstick cooking spray, set aside. Beat margarine and maltitol until light and creamy. Beat in egg. Sift dry ingredients together. Add prunes and nuts to dry mixture, then add this mixture to batter. Blend in applesauce. Bake for 1 hour or until it is tests done. Let cool on rack in pan for 10 minutes before turning out of pan. Serve with sweetened whipped cream, if desired.

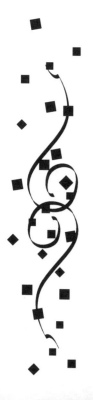

Chocolate Amaretto Mousse Cake

Serving Size: 12

6 ounces unsweetened chocolate squares, chopped
3/4 cup maltitol plus 2 tbsps
1/3 cup water
1/2 pound unsalted butter
4 eggs
2 tbsps amaretto (almond liqueur)

Preheat the oven to 300°F and butter a 8 inch round cake pan and line the bottom with a circle of parchment or wax paper, set aside.

Combine the chocolate, maltitol and water in a small saucepan over low heat and stir until chocolate is completely melted. Remove from the heat and stir in the butter until it is all melted. In another bowl, whip together the amaretto and eggs until it is smooth, then slowly pour in the chocolate mixture while whipping, continue to mix only until everything is combined. Pour the batter into the prepared pan and place it in a baking dish that is larger than the cake pan. Fill the baking dish with warm water so that it is 1/2 way up the side of the cake pan. Bake for about 45 minutes, until the cake is set. Remove the cake pan from the water bath and let it cool completely in the pan. When it is cool, cover it with plastic wrap and refrigerate it for about an hour to firm it up a little. To unmold the cake, run a knife around the inside to loosen the sides and dip the pan in hot water to loosen the bottom. Invert the cake onto a flat-bottomed plate and remove the paper. This cake is lovely garnished with toasted sliced almonds or a dusting of unsweetened cocoa powder.

Notes: This cake is very versatile in the fact that you can change the liqueurs being used to whatever you like (as long as it is good with chocolate). A few good choices are: hazelnut liqueur, orange liqueur, raspberry liqueur, creme de menthe, or dark rum.

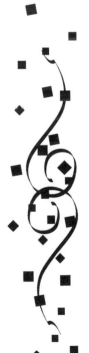

Chocolate Pound Cake

Serving Size: 10

3 ounces unsweetened chocolate squares, chopped
1 cup all-purpose flour
1/4 tsp baking powder
1/4 tsp baking soda
1/4 tsp salt
8 tbsps unsalted butter
1 cup maltitol
2 eggs
1/2 tsp vanilla extract
4 ounces lowfat sour cream

Preheat oven to 325°F and spray a 8 1/2X4 1/2X3 inch loaf pan with nonstick cooking spray, set aside. Place the chocolate in a small bowl over hot water and melt the chocolate, stirring occasionally, set aside to cool. Sift together flour, baking powder and soda and salt, set aside. Whip the butter until it is very fluffy and white, then gradually add maltitol while still mixing. Add chocolate to the butter mixture and combine well, them mix in sour cream. Add the flour mixture and beat until the mixture is smooth. Pour into prepared pan and bake about 45 minutes, or until a knife inserted in the center comes out clean. Cool the cake in the pan for 10 minutes, then turn out onto a rack to cool completely.

Notes: Serve chocolate pound cake with sweetened whipped cream and berries or sugarfree ice cream.

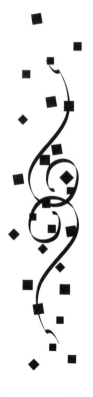

Chocolate Zucchini Cake

Serving Size: 12

2 1/2 cups all-purpose flour
1 cup unsweetened cocoa powder
1 tsp double-acting baking powder
1 tsp baking soda
1 tsp salt
1 tsp ground cinnamon
3/4 cup butter, softened
2 cups maltitol
3 eggs
3/4 cup lowfat buttermilk
1 tsp vanilla extract
2 tsps orange peel, grated
2 cups zucchini, shredded
1 cup pecans, chopped

Preheat oven to 350°F and spray a 10 inch tube pan with nonstick cooking spray, set aside. Sift together flour, cocoa, baking powder, baking soda, cinnamon, and salt. Cream butter. Gradually add maltitol, beat until fluffy. Add eggs one at a time, beating well after each. Beat in sifted dry ingredients, alternately with buttermilk. Stir in vanilla, orange peel, zucchini and nuts. Bake for one hour. Let cool for 15 minutes, turn out onto a rack to cool completely.

Notes: This cake is so divine, the only embellishment it needs is a dab of whipped cream.

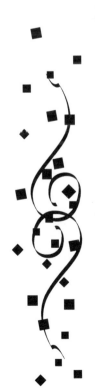

Quick Hints
Keeping a Cookbook Flat

To keep the open pages of a cookbook or magazine flat, readable and clean while cooking, put a clear glass (Pyrex) baking dish over it.

Fresh Apple Pound Cake

Serving Size: 20

3 cups flour
1 tsp baking soda
1 tsp salt
1 tsp cinnamon
1 tsp nutmeg
1 1/2 cup corn oil
2 cups maltitol
3 eggs
2 tsp vanilla
2 cups finely chopped, peeled apples
1 cup finely chopped pecans
1/2 cup unsweetened coconut

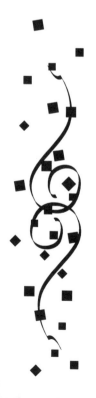

Preheat oven to 350°F. Prepare a 12 cup bundt pan with nonstick cooking spray. Combine flour, baking soda, salt, cinnamon and nutmeg. Set aside. Beat oil, maltitol, eggs and vanilla in large mixing bowl on medium speed until combined thoroughly. Add flour mixture; beat until smooth. Fold in apples, pecans and coconut. Turn into prepared pan. Bake 1 hour and 10 minutes or until done. Cool cake in pan on wire rack until complete cool. Remove from pan.

Orange and Sour Cream Cake

Serving Size: 16

1/3 cup unsalted butter
3 tbsps brown sugar replacement
2/3 cup maltitol
2 eggs
1 1/3 cups all-purpose flour
1/2 tsp baking soda
2 tsps double-acting baking powder
1/2 tsp salt
1 pint lowfat sour cream
2/3 cup skim milk
2 cups orange sections

Preheat oven to 350°F and spray a 13X9X2 inch baking dish with nonstick cooking spray. Cream butter and brown sugar replacement until light and fluffy. Gradually add in maltitol while mixing. Blend in vanilla. Beat in eggs one at a time. Stir flour, salt, soda, and baking powder together thoroughly; blend into creamed mixture alternately with 1/2 cup sour cream and milk. Begin and end with flour. Pour into prepared pan. Bake in 25-35 minutes or until done. Cool completely before removing from pan. Cut cake in half to form 2 layers 6-1/2 by 9 inches. Spread 3/4 cup sour cream over layer, arrange orange slices on sour cream. Top with second layer.

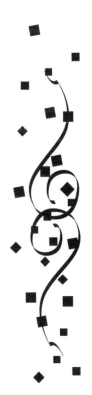

Pound Cake

Serving Size: 12

2 cups all-purpose flour
1 1/2 tsps baking powder
1 cup butter, softened
1 cup maltitol
1 tsp vanilla extract
4 eggs at room temperature

Preheat the oven to 350°F and spray a 9X5X3 inch loaf pan with nonstick cooking spray and set aside. Sift together flour and baking powder and set aside. Whip butter until white and fluffy, then slowly add maltitol and vanilla while beating. Add eggs one at a time, beating well after each addition. Add flour mixture to batter and mix just until combined. Pour batter into prepared pan and bake for one hour, or until a knife inserted in the middle comes out clean. Allow cake to cool in pan 10 minutes before turning it out onto a rack to cool completely before slicing.

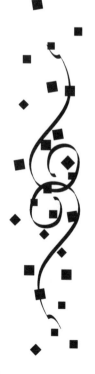

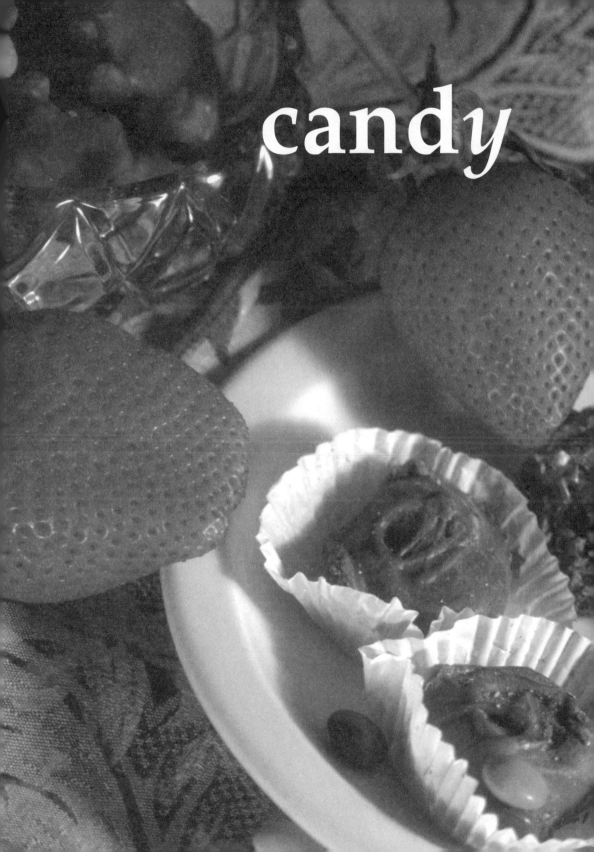

candy

Almond Balls

Serving Size: 20

1 cup all-purpose flour
1/2 cup margarine
1 cup almonds, ground
2 tbsps maltitol
1 tsp almond extract

Preheat oven to 375°F. Combine all ingredients in a large
bowl, mix thoroughly. Refrigerate dough for 30 minutes. Form
dough into 1-1/4 inch balls. Place 1 inch apart on ungreased
cookie sheet. Bake for 15-20 minutes or until set but not
brown. Let stand 1 minute in pan then remove to wire rack.

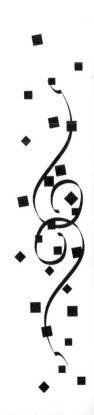

Chocolate Hazelnut Pretzels

Serving Size: 40

3 ounces unsweetened chocolate squares, chopped fine
1 1/2 cups all-purpose flour
3/4 cup ground hazelnuts
3/4 cup butter, softened
1/2 cup maltitol

Preheat oven to 375°F. Melt chocolate over a double boiler and set aside to cool. Whip butter until light and fluffy, then gradually add in maltitol while mixing. Combine hazelnut meal and flour. Add chocolate to butter mixture, then add in flour mixture. Make sure all ingredients are evenly combined. Divide dough in half and refrigerate it for at least 30 minutes, or until it is easier to handle. Pull off about 1 tablespoon of dough at a time, rolling each piece out 8 inches long. To shape the pretzel, cross one end over the other, leaving about 1 inch of the ends free. Lift ends to the opposite side of the pretzel and press down gently. Carefully lift the pretzels to an ungreased baking sheet. Repeat with remaining dough. Bake 6-8 minutes then transfer to a wire rack to cool.

Notes: Different nuts can be exchanged for hazelnuts, if desired.

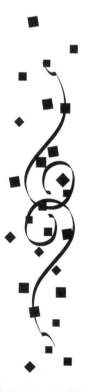

Grand Marnier Truffles

Serving Size: 20

1 cup heavy cream
3/4 cup maltitol
8 ounces unsweetened chocolate*
2 tbsps butter
2 tbsps Grand Marnier (orange liqueur)
1 tbsp orange zest, finely grated
Coating
2 ounces unsweetened chocolate, melted
4 tbsps maltitol

To make the filling for the truffles, combine the cream and maltitol in a saucepan and bring to a simmer over medium heat. Remove from the heat and add the chocolate and butter and whisk until smooth. Add the Grand Marnier and orange zest and stir until evenly distributed. Pour the chocolate mixture into a bowl and let it chill completely in the refrigerator (it should get pretty firm). Once the chocolate is firm, use a spoon or melon baller to scoop out balls that are 1-1 1/2 inch in diameter. If necessary, roll the balls between your palms to shape them. When all the balls are made, place them on a cookie sheet and refrigerate them again (you may want to slightly flatten one side of the truffle so it will stand up straight). While the truffle fillings are in the refrigerator firming up again, make the coating by combining the melted chocolate and maltitol. Keep the mixture slightly warm so that the coating will be flawless. One the coating is made, dip each truffle in the chocolate coating and place it on a pan covered in plastic to dry. You can repeat this step if desired. It is best to let the truffle coating harden up at room temperature. Store truffles covered at room temperature, or if you plan to keep them longer, in the refrigerator, tightly covered.

*Notes: It is best to use the very best unsweetened chocolate you can find because truffles are, in essence, a fancy hunk of chocolate, and if your chocolate does not have much flavor, neither will your truffles.

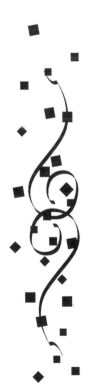

Hazelnut Truffles

Serving Size: 20

1 cup heavy cream
3/4 cup maltitol
8 ounces unsweetened chocolate
2 tbsps butter
3 tbsps hazelnut liqueur
1 cup hazelnuts
2 ounces unsweetened chocolate
4 tbsps maltitol

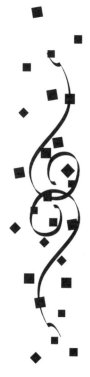

To make the filling for the truffles, combine the cream and maltitol in a saucepan and bring to a simmer over medium heat. Remove from the heat and add the chocolate and butter and whisk until smooth. Add the hazelnut liqueur and stir until evenly distributed. Pour the chocolate mixture into a bowl and let it chill completely in the refrigerator (it should get pretty firm). Once the chocolate is firm, use a spoon or melon baller to scoop out balls that are 1-1 1/2 inch in diameter. If necessary, roll the balls between your palms to shape them. When all the balls are made, place them on a cookie sheet and refrigerate them again (you may want to slightly flatten one side of the truffle so it will stand up straight). To get the hazelnuts ready for the truffles, preheat the oven to 350°F. Place the nuts on a baking sheet and toast them for about 8-10 minutes. If the nuts still have their skins on them, once they are done toasting, place them in a towel and rub them vigorously to remove the skin. Allow the nuts to cool off, then chop them very finely. While the truffle

continued on page 93

fillings are in the refrigerator firming up again, make the coating by combining the melted chocolate and maltitol. Keep the mixture slightly warm. One the coating is made, dip each truffle in the chocolate coating and roll it in the chopped hazelnuts. It is best to let the truffle coating harden up at room temperature. Store truffles covered at room temperature, or if you plan to keep them longer, in the refrigerator, tightly covered.

Notes: This same recipe can be used to make Amaretto Truffles - simply substitute almond liqueur for the hazelnut liqueur and chopped almonds for the hazelnuts.

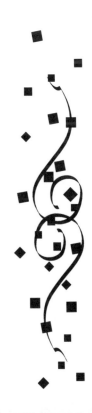

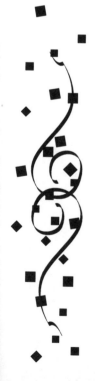

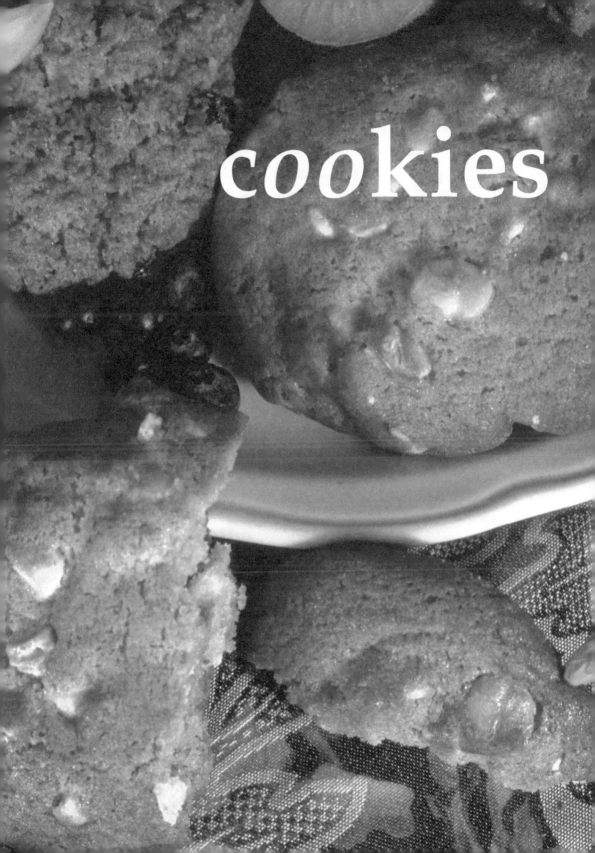

cookies

Apple Pie Squares

Serving Size: 24

2 1/2 cups all-purpose flour
1 tsp salt
1 cup shortening
1 egg yolk, beaten
milk
1 cup crushed cornflakes
10 medium cored Granny Smith apples, peeled &
    sliced thin
3/4 cup maltitol
1 tsp cinnamon

Preheat oven to 375°F. Combine flour and salt and cut in shortening with a pastry blender or two knives. Combine egg yolk and enough milk to make 1/3 cup and sprinkle it 1 tablespoon at a time over the flour mixture until a dough can be formed. Roll out half the dough into a 15X10 inch rectangle and place it in a pan of the same size. Sprinkle crushed cornflakes over the bottom crust. Combine apples, syrup and cinnamon and spread over the crushed cereal. Roll out the remaining dough and place it on top of the apples, sealing the edges. Prick the top dough . Bake about an hour or until golden. Cool in pan then cut into squares when it is room temperature. Store bars in the refrigerator.

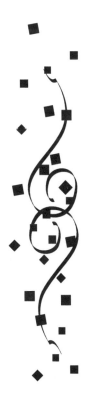

Apricot Almond Bars

Serving Size: 36

1 cup dried apricots
1/2 cup toasted almonds, ground
1/2 cup soft butter
1/4 cup maltitol
1 cup all-purpose flour
1/2 tsp baking powder
1/4 tsp salt
2 eggs
1/2 cup brown sugar replacement
1/2 cup maltitol
1/2 tsp vanilla extract
1/4 tsp almond extract

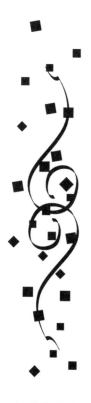

Preheat oven to 350°F. Place apricots in a small sauce pan and cover them with water. Bring to a boil over medium high heat, cover and simmer about 8 minutes, or until tender. Drain and pat dry with paper towels. Cut apricots into thin slivers, set aside. Whip butter until it is light and fluffy, then gradually add maltitol. Add the ground almonds and 1/2 cup of the flour. Spread this mixture into the bottom of an ungreased 9 inch square baking dish and bake for 20 minutes, set aside to cool. While the crust is baking, combine the remaining 1/2 cup of flour, baking powder and salt, set aside. Beat eggs until pale in color then add brown sugar replacement and maltitol gradually. Add flour mixture a little at a time, then blend in extracts. Stir in apricots then spread the mixture over the baked layer. Return the dish to the oven and bake about 30 minutes more, or until well browned. Cut into squares and remove bars from pan after they have cooled completely.

Apricot Bars

Serving Size: 24

1/2 cup dried apricots, finely chopped
1/2 cup golden raisins
1/3 cup water
1 cup all-purpose flour
1 tsp baking powder
1/4 tsp baking soda
1/2 cup almonds, chopped
1/2 cup crushed pineapple
2 large eggs
1 tbsp lemon juice
1 cup maltitol

Preheat oven to 350°F. Place apricots and raisins in a saucepan; cover with water. Simmer for 8 to 10 minutes or until tender. Drain well. Combine flour, baking powder and baking soda. Add chopped nuts, drained pineapple and drained cooked fruit to dry ingredients. Stir just enough to coat with flour. Beat eggs with lemon juice until just foamy. Gradually add maltitol, beating until just blended. Fold into the flour mixture. Spread in a 9-inch pan that has been sprayed with nonstick cooking spray. Bake for 35 to 40 minutes or until golden brown. While still warm, cut into bars.

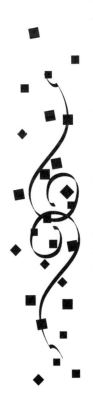

Apricot Squares

Serving Size: 16

3/4 cup dried apricots
1 cup water
1/2 cup butter
1/4 cup maltitol
1 1/3 cups all-purpose flour
1/2 tsp baking powder
1 cup brown sugar replacement
2 large eggs

Preheat oven to 350°F and spray a 8 inch square baking dish with nonstick cooking spray, set aside. Place apricots and 1 cup water into a saucepan. Bring to a boil, reduce heat and simmer 10-15 minutes until apricots are tender. Drain and let cool. Fit steel knife blade into the work bowl of a food processor. Into the work bowl combine butter, maltitol and 1 cup flour. Process until smooth. Spread into the bottom of the prepared baking dish. Bake 25 minutes. With steel knife still attached, process drained apricots until chopped into small pieces. Add 1/3 cup flour, baking powder, brown sugar replacement and eggs. Process until mixed well, about 6-8 seconds. Remove crust from oven, spread apricot mixture evenly over baked crust and return to oven for 30 minutes longer. Let cool, then cut into 2-inch squares.

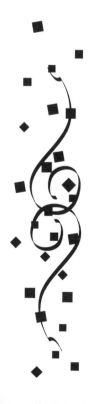

Blondies

Serving Size: 16

1/2 cup butter
1 cup brown sugar replacement
1 cup maltitol
2 eggs, beaten slightly
1 tbsp vanilla extract
1 cup all-purpose flour
2 tsps double-acting baking powder
1/2 tsp salt

Preheat oven to 350°F and spray a 9 inch square pan with nonstick cooking spray, set aside. Melt butter in saucepan. Stir brown sugar replacement and maltitol into butter until dissolved. Cool slightly and beat in egg and vanilla. Sift flour with baking powder and salt. Stir dry ingredients into butter mixture. Pour batter into pan. Bake for 30-45 minutes. Cool blondies completely before cutting.

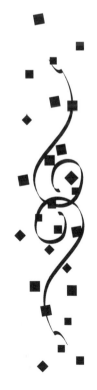

Brownies

Serving Size: 16

2 ounces unsweetened chocolate squares
1/4 cup butter
1 cup maltitol
1 egg
1 dash salt
1/2 cup all-purpose flour
1/2 cup chopped pecans
1 tsp vanilla extract

Preheat oven to 300°F. Spray an 8 inch square pan with nonstick cooking spray. Combine chocolate and butter in a sauce pot over low heat and stir until both are melted. Remove from heat and stir in maltitol, egg, salt, flour, pecans and vanilla, mixing just until combined. Spread into pan and bake for 30 minutes. Cool completely before cutting.

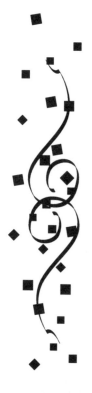

Cherry Fig Bars

Serving Size: 24

1 1/2 cups all-purpose flour
3/4 cup maltitol
1/2 cup soft butter
2 eggs, well beaten
1/2 tsp baking soda
1 tsp vanilla extract
3/4 cup chopped figs
1/4 cup chopped sweet cherries

Preheat oven to 325°F and spray a 9 inch square baking dish with nonstick cooking spray, set aside. Combine first 6 ingredients in a mixer bowl and mix until no traces of flour are left, about 2 minutes, then fold in figs and cherries. Spread the mixture into the prepared pan and bake for about 25 minutes, or until a toothpick inserted in the center comes out clean. Cool completely before cutting.

Notes: Use cherries that are packed in water or juice and drain them before chopping them.

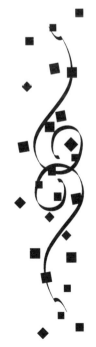

Coconut-Pineapple Bars

Serving Size: 36

1/2 cup soft butter
3/4 cup maltitol
1 1/4 cups all-purpose flour
1 1/4 pounds crushed pineapple, well drained
1 large egg
1 tbsp melted butter
1/2 tsp vanilla extract
3 1/2 ounces dried coconut, unsweetened

Preheat oven to 350°F. Combine 1/2 cup softened margarine and 1/4 cup maltitol in a small bowl. Beat with an electric mixer set on medium speed until mixture is light and fluffy. Gradually beat in flour to form a soft dough. Press dough evenly on bottom and 1/2 inch up sides of 9X9X1-3/4 inch ungreased pan. Bake for 15 minutes or until golden brown. Let cool. Spread pineapple over crust. Add remaining maltitol to egg; beat until just blended. Add 1 tablespoon melted butter, vanilla and coconut. Spread mixture over pineapple. Bake 20 minutes longer, or until top is golden brown. Cool, then cut into 1-1/2 inch squares.

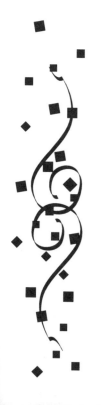

Coffee Almond Bars

Serving Size: 36

2 1/4 cups all-purpose flour
3/4 cup maltitol
1 cup butter or margarine, softened
1 egg
1 1/2 tsps instant coffee granules
1 cup sliced almonds, lightly toasted

Preheat oven to 350°F. Spray a 9X13X2 inch baking dish with nonstick cooking spray and set aside. Combine all ingredients, except almonds, and mix for about 3 minutes, scraping the sides and the bottom of the bowl frequently. Stir in almonds by hand, then press mixture into the bottom of the prepared pan. Bake for about 25 minutes, or until the edges turn golden brown. Allow to cool completely in pan before cutting into bars.

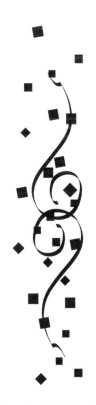

Cottage Cheese Squares

Serving Size: 8

1 recipe sweet tart dough *(recipe on page 265)*
2 cups nonfat cottage cheese
1 cup nonfat ricotta cheese
1 tbsp melted butter
3 tbsps maltitol
2 tbsps grated orange rind
1 tsp orange juice
1/4 tsp cinnamon

Preheat oven to 325°F and roll out tart dough 1/4 inch thick. Line the bottom of an 8 inch square dish with the dough and bake it for 15 minutes, set aside to cool. Reduce heat to 300°F. In a blender or food processor, puree cottage cheese, ricotta, butter, maltitol, orange rind, orange juice and cinnamon. Pour into prepared pan and bake until firm (about 25 minutes). Remove from oven and let cool, then slice into squares. Serve chilled.

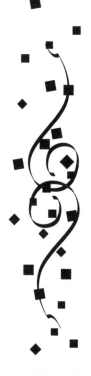

Cream Cheese and Peanut Butter Surprises

Serving Size: 30

1 cup all-purpose flour
2 tbsps maltitol
1/2 tsp salt
1/3 cup vegetable shortening
3 ounces lowfat cream cheese, softened
2 tsps skim milk
1/4 cup peanut butter, no sugar added
3 tbsps apple butter, no sugar added

Preheat oven to 400°F and spray cookie sheet(s) with nonstick cooking spray. In a small mixing bowl, sift the flour with maltitol and salt. Add shortening, cream cheese and milk. Mix on lowest speed of an electric mixer until dough begins to form. Shape into a ball. Roll out on floured surface to a 20 x 8 inch rectangle. Cut in half to make two 10 x 8-inch rectangles.

Spread one half with peanut butter; top with the apple butter. Place the second half of dough on top of first. Brush with milk. Cut into strips 5 x 1/2 inches. Gently twist twice. Place on cookie sheets and bake for 7-10 minutes or until light golden brown. Makes 30 twists.

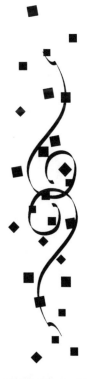

Cream Cheese Marbled Brownies

Serving Size: 18

Cream Cheese Mixture:
2 tbsps soft margarine
3 ounces lowfat cream cheese
1/4 cup maltitol
1 egg, well beaten
1 tbsp all-purpose flour
1/2 tsp vanilla extract
Brownie Mixture:
2 ounces unsweetened chocolate squares, chopped fine
3 tbsps margarine
1/2 cup all-purpose flour
1/2 tsp baking powder
1/4 tsp salt
2 eggs
1 cup maltitol
1/2 tsp vanilla extract
1/2 cup chopped nuts, optional

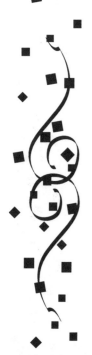

Preheat oven to 350°F and spray an 8 inch square baking dish with nonstick cooking spray, set aside. To make cream cheese mixture, combine margarine and cream cheese and mix until soft and well blended. Add maltitol, mix well. Add egg, mix well. Add flour, mix well. Add vanilla, mix well and set mixture aside.

continued on page 109

To make brownies, combine chocolate and butter in a small saucepan over low heat. Let mixture stand until both items are melted, then stir smooth. Set aside to cool. Stir together flour, baking powder and salt, set aside. Beat eggs at high speed until they are light colored, then gradually beat in maltitol and vanilla. Gradually add flour mixture, beating until thoroughly combined. Stir in chocolate mixture until batter is well combined. Add nuts, if desired. Pour half of batter into prepared baking dish, then top it with the cream cheese mixture (spread the cheese mixture to the edges of the pan). Pour the remaining brownie mixture on top and swirl a thin spatula through the layers to create a marbled effect, if desired. Bake for about 40 minutes, or until the brownies pull away from the edges of the pan. Cool completely before cutting into bars.

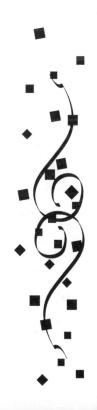

Crunchy Chocolate-Nut Bars

Serving Size: 24

Crust:
1/2 cup butter
1/2 cup brown sugar replacement
1 egg yolk
1 tsp vanilla extract
1/2 cup all-purpose flour
1/2 cup rolled oats, not instant
Topping:
2 ounces unsweetened chocolate squares
1/4 cup maltitol
1 tbsp butter
1/2 cup sliced almonds, toasted

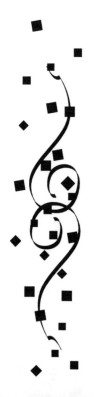

Preheat oven to 375°F. Spray a 13X9X2 inch pan with nonstick cooking spray. To prepare crust, beat butter, brown sugar replacement, egg yolk, and vanilla until smooth, using an electric mixer. Add flour and oats; stir until well combined. Press mixture into the bottom of prepared pan. Bake for 15 minutes or until golden brown. Cool slightly. To make topping, melt chocolate, maltitol and butter over hot, not boiling, water. Spread over warm cookie crust. Sprinkle evenly with sliced almonds. While still warm, cut into bars using a sharp knife. Let cool completely before removing from pan.

Dream Bars

Serving Size: 36

Crust:
1 cup all-purpose flour
1/3 cup maltitol
1/2 cup soft butter
 Filling:
1 cup maltitol
1/4 cup peanut butter, no sugar added
2 eggs, well beaten
1/2 tsp vanilla extract
1/2 cup unsweetened shredded coconut
1/2 cup malt-sweetened chocolate chips

Preheat oven to 350°F and spray a 9 inch square baking pan
with nonstick cooking spray. To make crust, combine all crust
ingredients and mix until no traces of flour are left, about 2
minutes. Press onto the bottom of the prepared pan and bake
for about 15 minutes, or until the edges are lightly browned.
Set aside to cool.

For the filling, combine everything except chocolate chips and
mix until well combined. Stir in chocolate chips by hand. Pour
mixture over crust and bake for about 25 minutes, or until
filling is set and light brown. Cool completely before cutting
into bars.

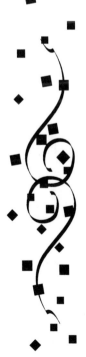

Honey Bunny Bars

Serving Size: 48

3/4 cup butter
1 cup maltitol, honey flavored
1 large egg, beaten
1/2 tsp salt
1 cup mashed bananas, ripe
1 tsp vanilla extract
1/2 cup creamy peanut butter, no sugar added
4 cups rolled oats

Preheat oven to 350°F and spray a 13X9X2 inch pan with nonstick cooking spray, set aside. Cream the butter and maltitol until light and fluffy. Add the beaten egg, salt, bananas, vanilla and peanut butter. Beat until very well mixed. Stir in the oats and blend thoroughly. Spread the mixture evenly in pan. Bake for 50-60 minutes or until a toothpick inserted in center comes out clean. Cool slightly, then cut into bars of about 1 x 2 inches.

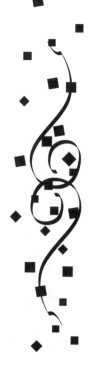

Honey Carrot Bars

Serving Size: 36

1 1/2 cups all-purpose flour
1 cup melted butter
1 cup maltitol, honey flavored
3 eggs, well beaten
1 1/2 tsps baking soda
1 tsp cinnamon
1/2 tsp salt
1 1/2 cups shredded carrots
3/4 cup chopped pecans
Icing, optional
1/2 cup maltitol
8 ounces lowfat cream cheese, softened
1 tsp vanilla extract

Preheat oven to 350°F and spray a 15X10 inch pan with nonstick cooking spray, set aside. To make the bars, combine all ingredients and mix for about 3 minutes, or until everything is well blended. Pour into prepared pan and bake for about 20 minutes, or until top springs back when touched lightly. Set aside to cool completely.

To make the icing, blend the cream cheese until it is very soft, then gradually add maltitol and vanilla and mix until there are no lumps. Spread over bars that have completely cooled off.

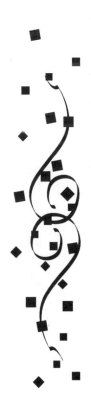

Lemon Squares

Serving Size: 16

Crust:
1/3 cup butter
1/4 cup maltitol
1 cup all-purpose flour
Topping:
2 eggs
1/2 cup maltitol
2 tbsps all-purpose flour
1 tbsp lemon zest, grated
3 tbsps fresh lemon juice
1/4 tsp baking powder

Preheat oven to 350°F. Whip butter on high speed for one minute, then gradually add maltitol. Add flour and mix until crumbly. Press into bottom of 8 inch square pan and bake for about 16 minutes, or until it is golden.

While crust is baking, combine all remaining ingredients and mix until completely combined. Pour over hot, baked crust then bake for about 20 minutes more, or until center is set. Allow bars to cool completely before cutting.

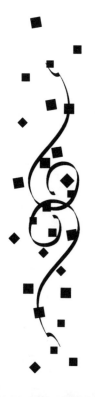

Mocha Chip Bars

Serving Size: 16

1/2 cup butter
1/2 cup brown sugar replacement
1 1/4 cups maltitol
2 egg
1 tsp vanilla extract
1 tbsp instant coffee
1/2 tsp salt
2 cups all-purpose flour
2 tsps double-acting baking powder
1 cup sliced almonds
1 cup malt sweetened chocolate chips

Preheat oven to 350°F and spray a 13X9X2 inch pan with nonstick cooking spray, set aside. Cream butter, brown sugar replacement, and maltitol together until light and fluffy. Beat in eggs and vanilla. Sift dry ingredients and coffee together and add to egg mixture. Stir in chocolate chips and nuts. Pour batter into pan. Bake for 20 minutes. Allow bars to cool completely before cutting.

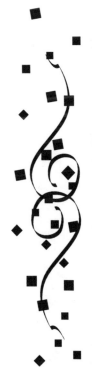

Orange Bars

Serving Size: 36

1/4 cup flour
1/2 tsp baking powder
2 eggs
1/2 cup brown sugar replacement
1/2 cup maltitol
1 tsp vanilla extract
1 tbsp grated orange peel
1 cup chopped almonds
1 1/2 cups flaked coconut, unsweetened
Pastry:
1/2 cup butter softened
1/2 cup maltitol
1 tsp grated orange peel
1 cup flour

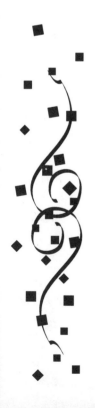

Preheat oven to 375°F and spray a 13X9X2 inch baking pan with nonstick cooking spray. Prepare orange pastry: in mixer bowl combine butter, maltitol, and orange peel, beat until fluffy. Gradually stir in flour until mixture is well combined (dough will be crumbly). Press firmly and evenly over bottom of baking pan. Bake for 10 minutes, then remove pastry from oven. Reduce temperature to 350°F. In a small bowl combine flour and baking powder; stir to combine thoroughly. In mixer bowl combine eggs, brown sugar replacement and maltitol, beat until well mixed. Blend in vanilla and orange peel. Gradually beat in flour mixture until well combined. Stir in almonds and coconut. Spread mixture over partially baked pastry. Bake until well browned and set in center, about 20 to 25 minutes. Remove pan to a rack. Let stand about 5 minutes, then cut into bars. Remove from pan when cool.

Orange-Prune Bars

Serving Size: 24

Crust
1/2 cup butter, softened
1/2 cup brown sugar replacement
1 cup all-purpose flour
Filling
1 1/4 cups dried prunes
1/3 cup brown sugar replacement
2 tbsps cornstarch
1/8 tsp salt
1/4 cup orange juice
1 tbsp orange zest, grated
1 cup walnuts
2 large eggs
3 1/2 ounces dried coconut, unsweetened

Preheat oven to 350°F. To make crust, place softened butter and brown sugar replacement in small bowl. With electric mixer set on medium speed, cream mixture until light and fluffy. Turn mixer to low and beat in flour. Mixture will be creamy. Pat dough evenly into bottom of 9 x 9 x 1-3/4 inch ungreased pan. Bake for 10-12 minutes, or until golden brown. Let cool 15-20 minutes. To make filling, place prunes into a saucepan with just enough water to cover. Cook over medium heat for 30 minutes. Drain and reserve 2 tablespoons of the liquid. Cut prunes into 4-5 pieces, removing pits. Combine prunes in saucepan with reserved 2 tablespoons liquid, brown sugar substitute, cornstarch, salt, orange juice and zest. Bring to a boil; reduce heat and simmer, stirring constantly, for 2-3 minutes or until thickened. Stir in coarsely chopped walnuts, spread over crust. Place the eggs in a small bowl and beat until frothy. Stir in the coconut. Spread evenly over prune mixture. Bake 25 minutes. Cool slightly and cut into 24 bars.

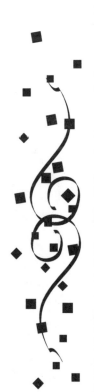

Peanutty Chocolate Chip Bars

Serving Size: 60

1/2 cup brown sugar replacement
3/4 cup maltitol
1 cup soft butter
1 egg, well beaten
1 tsp vanilla extract
2 1/4 cups all-purpose flour
1 tsp baking soda
1/2 tsp salt
1 cup chopped peanuts
1 cup malt sweetened chocolate chips
 Topping:
1 cup malt sweetened chocolate chips
1/2 cup peanut butter, no sugar added
1/2 cup chopped peanuts

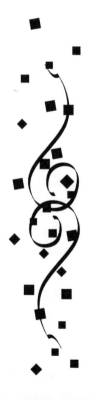

Preheat oven to 375°F. Combine brown sugar replacement, maltitol, butter, egg and vanilla and mix until well combined. Scrape down sides and bottom. Add flour, baking soda and salt and mix until no traces of flour are left. Stir in peanuts and chocolate chips by hand. Press evenly into the bottom of a 15X10 inch jelly roll pan and bake for about 15 minutes, or until the edges begin to brown.

To make the topping, combine the chocolate chips and peanut butter in a small sauce pan over low heat and stir until chips have melted. Spread this mixture over the warm bars then sprinkle the peanuts over the top. Refrigerate for an hour before cutting into bars.

Pecan Raspberry Bars

Serving Size: 24

2 1/4 cups all-purpose flour
1 cup maltitol
1 cup chopped pecans
1 cup soft butter
1 egg, well beaten
10 ounces all-fruit raspberry preserves, no sugar added

Preheat oven to 350°F and spray an 8 inch square pan with nonstick cooking spray, set aside. Combine all ingredients, except preserves, in a bowl and mix for about 2 minutes, or until everything is well combined. Set aside 1 1/2 cups of the mixture and press the remaining into the bottom of the prepared pan. Stir the preserves so that they are spreadable and spread them to within 1/2 inch of the edges. Sprinkle the reserved mixture over the top then bake for about 45 minutes, or until lightly browned. Cool completely before cutting into bars.

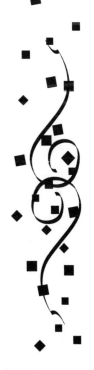

Strawberry Bars

Serving Size: 36

Crust:
1 1/2 cups all-purpose flour
1/2 cup quick-cooking oats
1/2 cup maltitol
3/4 cup soft butter
1/2 tsp baking soda
Topping:
3/4 cup unsweetened shredded coconut
3/4 cup chopped almonds
1/4 cup all-purpose flour
1/4 cup brown sugar replacement
2 tbsps soft butter
10 ounces strawberry all-fruit preserves, no sugar
    added

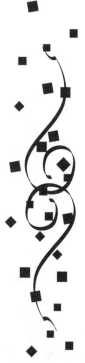

Preheat oven to 350°F and spray a 13X9 inch baking dish with nonstick cooking spray, set aside. Combine all crust ingredients and mix until no traces of flour are left and mixture is combined well. Press into the bottom of the prepared pan and bake about 20 minutes, or until the edges begin to brown. For the topping, combine all except the preserves, and mix until combined well, scraping the bowl often, set aside. Stir the preserves until they are easily spread and spread them over the hot crust within 1/4 inch of the edge. Sprinkle topping mixture over the top of the preserves. Bake for about 20 minutes more or until light brown. Cool completely before cutting into bars.

Almond Chocolate Sandwich Cookies

Serving Size: 48

8 tbsps unsalted butter, softened
1/2 cup maltitol
2 egg whites
1/4 cup all-purpose flour
2 tbsps unsweetened cocoa powder
1 cup ground almonds
1/2 cup heavy cream
3 ounces unsweetened chocolate squares, chopped
3 tbsps maltitol

Preheat oven to 350°F and lightly spray cookie sheet(s) with nonstick cooking spray, set aside. Whip the butter until it is very fluffy and white, then gradually add maltitol and egg whites. Scrape bowl. Sift together cocoa powder and flour and stir into the mixture. Stir in ground almonds. Place rounded teaspoons of dough on the prepared sheets and bake for 8-10 minutes, or until they are firm. To make filling, heat the cream and maltitol until very hot but not boiling. Add chopped chocolate and stir until smooth. To assemble cookies, take one cookie and spread some of the chocolate mixture on the flat side of the cookie with a spoon. Top that cookie with the flat side of another cookie and press them together slightly. Repeat until all the cookies are used.

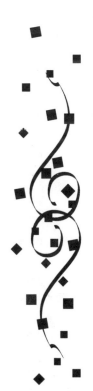

Almond Shortbread

Serving Size: 30

2 cups all-purpose flour
1 cup maltitol
1 cup soft butter
1 egg separated
1/2 tsp almond extract
1 tbsp milk
1/2 cup chopped almonds

Preheat oven to 350°F and spray a 15X10 inch jelly roll pan with nonstick cooking spray, set aside. Combine flour, maltitol, butter, egg yolk and extract in a bowl and mix until well combined. Press onto the bottom of the prepared pan. In a separate bowl, mix the egg white and the milk until it is a little frothy then brush it onto the top of the dough. Sprinkle the nuts over the dough and press them down lightly with your hands. Bake for about 15-20 minutes, or until very light brown. Cool completely before cutting.

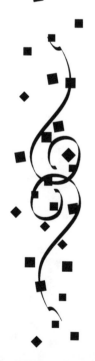

Anise Cookies

Serving Size: 48

3 cups all-purpose flour
1 1/2 tsps baking powder
1 tsp crushed anise seed
1 cup soft margarine
3/4 cup maltitol
1/2 tsp vanilla extract
1 egg
2 tbsps brandy

Preheat oven to 350°F and spray cookie sheet(s) with nonstick cooking spray, set aside. Combine flour, baking powder and anise, set aside. Whip butter until fluffy and gradually add maltitol. Add vanilla, egg and brandy and beat well. Add flour mixture and mix well. Shape dough into 1 inch balls and place them on prepared cookie sheets. Dip a flat bottomed glass in water and flatten the cookies to 1/4 inch thickness with it. Bake cookies about 10 minutes or until the edges are slightly browned.

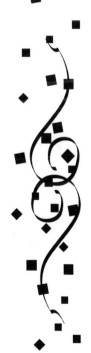

Apple Pecan Spice Cookies

Serving Size: 48

1 3/4 cups all-purpose flour
1 tsp baking soda
1 tsp cinnamon
1/4 tsp nutmeg
1/4 tsp allspice
1/2 cup soft butter
1/2 cup brown sugar replacement
1 cup maltitol
1 egg
1/4 cup apple juice, no sugar added
1 large apple, chopped
1 cup chopped pecans

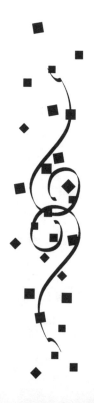

Preheat oven to 400°F and lightly spray cookie sheet(s) with nonstick cooking spray, set aside. Sift together first 5 ingredients, set aside. Whip butter and brown sugar replacement until it is very fluffy, then gradually add maltitol while mixing. Add egg, mix well, then apple juice. Add flour mixture to the butter mixture and mix for about 3 minutes, or until everything is well combined. Add apple and pecans and mix until they are evenly dispersed in the batter. Drop cookies by teaspoonfuls onto prepared cookie sheet and bake for about 10 minutes, or until lightly browned.

Apricot Raisin Cookies

Serving Size: 72

1 cup seedless raisins
1 cup dried apricots, minced
1 cup shortening
1 3/4 cups maltitol
2 eggs
1 tsp vanilla extract
3 1/2 cups all-purpose flour
1 tsp double-acting baking powder
1 tsp baking soda
3/4 tsp salt
1/2 tsp ground cinnamon
1/2 tsp ground nutmeg
1/2 cup pecans, chopped

Cut the dried apricots into very small pieces; combine with the raisins and 1 cup water in a saucepan with lid. Bring to a boil and simmer, covered, for 3-4 minutes. Remove from heat, leave covered and allow to cool. Do not drain. In a mixing bowl, cream the shortening and add the maltitol gradually. Add the slightly beaten eggs and vanilla. Combine all the dry ingredients. Slowly add to egg mixture and blend thoroughly. Stir in the raisins, apricots and nuts. Drop by teaspoonfuls on cookie sheets that have been sprayed with nonstick cooking spray, 2 inches apart. Bake in preheated 350°F oven 12-14 minutes. Remove from cookie sheets and let cool on wire racks. Yield: about 6 dozen.

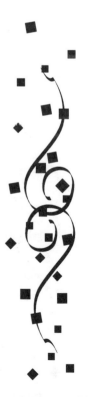

Banana Cookies

Serving Size: 36

1/2 cup soft butter
2 1/4 cups all-purpose flour
3/4 cup maltitol
2 eggs
1 tsp baking powder
1/4 tsp baking soda
1/2 tsp cinnamon
1/8 tsp allspice
1 cup mashed bananas
1/2 cup chopped pecans

Preheat oven to 375°F and spray cookie sheet(s) with nonstick cooking spray. Whip butter until very light and fluffy, then gradually mix in maltitol, then eggs, adding one at a time. Sift together flour, baking powder and soda, cinnamon and allspice. Add flour mixture alternately with mashed bananas to butter mixture until all ingredients are well blended. Stir in pecans. Drop by tablespoons onto prepared cookie sheets and bake for 10-12 minutes, or until edges are a light golden brown. Cool cookies 5 minutes on sheet before removing to cool completely.

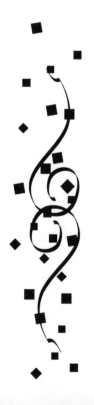

Banana Oatmeal Cookies

Serving Size: 72

1 cup maltitol
2/3 cup butter
2 eggs
3/4 cup mashed bananas
1/2 tsp vanilla
1/2 tsp lemon juice
1 1/2 cups rolled oats
2 cups flour
3/4 tsp baking soda
1 tsp baking powder
1 tsp salt
1/2 cup pecans

Sift flour, soda, baking powder and salt together. Cream together maltitol and shortening. Beat in well beaten eggs. Stir in the vanilla, lemon juice, and banana. Add rolled oats and nuts to flour mixture, alternately with banana mixture, mixing well after each addition. Stir in pecans. Drop by teaspoonfuls onto greased baking sheet and bake in preheated 350°F oven 15 to 18 minutes, or until golden.

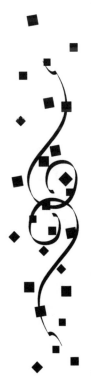

Banana Sandwich Cookies

Serving Size: 24

2 1/3 cups all-purpose flour
1 cup maltitol
1 cup soft butter
1/2 cup banana slices
1 tsp vanilla
1/2 cup chopped pecans
1/2 recipe banana buttercream, soft *(recipe on page 267)*

Preheat oven to 350°F and spray cookie sheet(s) with nonstick cooking spray, set aside. To make cookies, combine all ingredients (except buttercream) and mix until well blended, about 3 minutes. Scoop out dough by teaspoonfuls and shape them into a ball. Place the balls on prepared cookie sheets about 2 inches from each other and press them out to 1/4-inch thickness with the bottom of a glass dipped in water. Bake cookies for about 13 minutes, or until they are light brown. Remove from pan immediately and set aside to cool completely before icing.

When cookies are cool, spread about 2 teaspoons of the buttercream onto the flat side of a cookie and place another cookie on top of the icing. Press together slightly to make sure cookies stick. Repeat until all cookies are used.

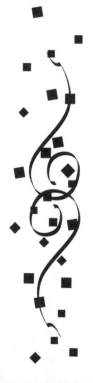

Quick Hints
Decorating Cookies
> *A gadget that works well for decorating sugar cookies is an empty plastic thread spool. Simply press the thread spool firmly into the cookie dough, imprinting the dough with a unique flower design.*

Brown Sugar Shortbread

Serving Size: 32

1/2 cup soft butter
2/3 cup brown sugar substitute
1/2 tsp vanilla extract
1 1/4 cups all-purpose flour

Preheat oven to 325°F and lightly spray a 9 inch square baking dish with nonstick cooking spray, set aside. Combine butter and brown sugar replacement in a bowl and beat until very fluffy. Blend in vanilla. Gradually add flour and stir until it is completely absorbed. Pat the dough evenly into the prepared pan. Bake for about 30 minutes or until the top feels firm. Let cookies cook in pan for 10 minutes then cut into 16 squares. Cut each square in half to make triangles. Remove from pan when completely cool.

Butter Cookies

Serving Size: 48

1 cup unsalted butter, softened
2/3 cup maltitol
2 tsps vanilla extract
2 cups flour
1/4 tsp salt

Preheat oven to 350°F. In large bowl of electric mixer, cream butter, maltitol, and vanilla until light and fluffy. Mix in flour and salt. Pat mixture evenly into an ungreased 10- by 15-inch jelly roll pan. Bake until pale in color, but not browned, about 16 to 18 minutes. Cool about 5 minutes, then cut into squares while still warm.

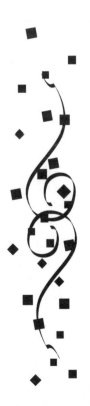

Cashew Cookies

Serving Size: 48

1/2 cup margarine
1/2 cup brown sugar replacement
1/2 cup maltitol
1 tsp baking powder
1/4 tsp baking soda
1 egg
1 tsp lemon zest, minced
2 tbsps fresh lemon juice
1 tsp vanilla extract
1 3/4 cups all-purpose flour
1 cup ground cashews
1/2 cup chopped cashews

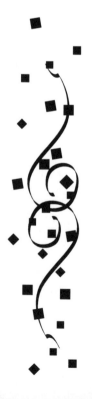

Preheat oven to 350°F. Whip butter until light and fluffy then gradually add brown sugar substitute and maltitol while mixing. Ad the egg and mix well. Combine baking powder and soda, lemon zest, flour and ground and chopped cashews. Add lemon juice and vanilla to the margarine mixture and beat well. Add flour mixture to margarine mixture and mix until no traces of flour are left. Drop dough in teaspoonfuls onto ungreased cookie sheet 2 inches apart from each other. Bake 10-12 minutes or until edges are lightly browned. Cool on sheet for one minute then transfer to wire rack to finish cooling.

Notes: Be sure to use unsalted cashews for this recipe.

Chinese Almond Cookies

Serving Size: 42

2 cups all-purpose flour
1/2 tsp baking powder
1 cup soft butter
1 cup maltitol
1 tsp almond extract
2 egg yolks
1/3 cup whole blanched almonds
2 tsps water

Preheat oven to 350°F and lightly spray cookie sheet(s) with nonstick cooking spray, set aside. Combine flour and baking powder, set aside. Whip butter until light and fluffy, then gradually add maltitol. Add almond extract and 1 egg yolk and beat well. Add flour mixture and blend well. Shape dough into 1 inch balls and place them on the prepared cookie sheet. Flatten each cookie slightly with your fingers then place an almond in the center. Beat the remaining egg yolk and water together. Brush the top of each cookie with the mixture. Bake cookies about 15 minutes or until they are golden brown. Let them sit on the cookie sheet for 2 minutes before removing them to a rack to cool completely.

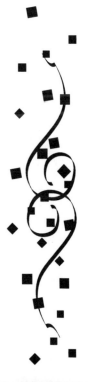

Chocolate Chip Oatmeal Cookies

Serving Size: 40

3/4 cup shortening
1 cup maltitol
1 egg
1 cup all-purpose flour
1/2 tsp baking soda
1/2 tsp baking powder
1/4 tsp salt
3 cups quick-cooking oats
1 1/2 cups malt sweetened chocolate chips
3/4 cup pecans, optional

Preheat oven to 350°F and spray cookie sheet(s) with nonstick cooking spray. Combine shortening, maltitol and egg and blend at medium speed until combined thoroughly. Combine flour, baking soda and powder and salt and add to butter mixture, stirring just until mixed. Add oats, chocolate chips and pecans, and stir in with a spoon. Drop by tbsps onto the greased cookie sheet, about 2 inch apart from each other. Bake about 14 minutes or until golden brown. Cool 5 minutes on cookie sheet before removing to cool completely.

Notes: Malt sweetened chocolate chips can be found at natural food stores.

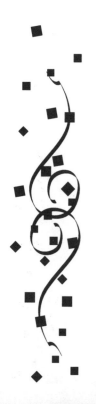

Chocolate Cinnamon Cookies

Serving Size: 36

2 cups all-purpose flour
2 tsps baking soda
1 tsp cinnamon
1/4 tsp salt
1/2 cup soft butter
1/4 cup shortening
1 1/4 cups maltitol
1 egg
2 ounces unsweetened chocolate squares, melted and
    cooled

Preheat oven to 350°F. Stir together flour, baking soda, cinnamon and salt, set aside. Combine butter and shortening and whip until light and fluffy. Gradually add the maltitol, beat well. Add the egg, beat well. Add the melted chocolate, beat well. Add the flour mixture and mix until no particles of flour are visible. Shape dough into balls that are about 1 inch and place on an ungreased cookie sheet about 2 inches apart from each other. Bake for about 15 minutes, or until cookies feel firm when lightly touched. Allow cookies to sit on cookie sheet 3 minutes before removing to a rack to finish cooling.

Notes: Chocolate and cinnamon are two flavors that compliment each other immensely.

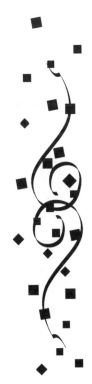

Chunky Raisin Cookies

Serving Size: 54

1 cup all-purpose flour
1 cup whole wheat flour
3/4 tsp baking soda
1 tsp cinnamon
1/4 tsp allspice
2/3 cup soft margarine
1/2 cup brown sugar replacement
1/2 cup maltitol
2 eggs, well beaten
1 1/2 cups raisins, soaked in hot water
1 cup chopped walnuts

Preheat oven to 350°F and lightly spray cookie sheet(s) with nonstick cooking spray, set aside. Sift together first 5 ingredients, set aside. Whip margarine until fluffy and add brown sugar replacement and whip one minute. With mixer on, gradually add maltitol and mix until it is well combined. Add eggs and mix well. Gradually add in flour mixture and mix until well blended. Remove raisins from hot water and squeeze out any excess water. Add the raisins and walnuts to the batter and mix until they are evenly dispersed. Drop by teaspoonfuls onto prepared pans and bake about 15 minutes, or until edges are browned.

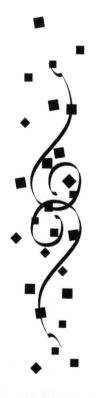

Cocoa Peanut Butter Cookies

Serving Size: 42

2/3 cup all-purpose flour
1/2 cup unsweetened cocoa powder
3/4 tsp baking powder
1/4 tsp baking soda
1/2 cup soft margarine
1/3 cup peanut butter, no sugar added
1 egg

Sift together first 4 ingredients, set aside. Combine margarine and peanut butter and beat to blend thoroughly. Add maltitol and blend well. Mix in egg. Gradually add flour mixture, mixing just until blended. Divide dough in half and place each on a sheet of plastic wrap. Shape each piece of dough into a log 2 inches across. Wrap each log tightly and refrigerate until firm, at least 2 hours. Preheat oven to 350°F. Cut logs into 1/4 inch slices, and arrange them on an ungreased cookie sheet 1 inch apart. Bake about 10 minutes, just until they are firm. Allow cookies to stand for 2 minutes before removing them to a rack to cool completely.

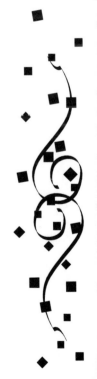

Coconut Drops

Serving Size: 60

2 cups all-purpose flour
1 tsp baking powder
1 tsp baking soda
1/2 tsp salt
1 cup quick-cooking oats
3 1/2 ounces dried coconut, unsweetened
3/4 cup vegetable shortening
3/4 cup maltitol
1/2 cup brown sugar replacement
1 tsp vanilla extract
1 large egg

Preheat oven to 375°F and lightly spray cookie sheet(s) with nonstick cooking spray. Sift flour, baking powder, baking soda and salt into a large bowl. Add the oats and coconut; set aside. Cream shortening with maltitol and brown sugar replacement until light and fluffy. Beat in vanilla and egg until well mixed. Gradually add flour mixture to make a stiff dough. Drop by teaspoonfuls, 1 inch apart, on prepared cookie sheets. Bake 10 minutes or until golden brown. Cool on cookie sheet for 5 minutes then remove to wire rack to cool completely.

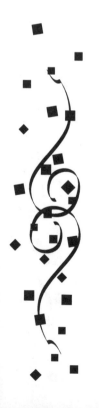

Coconut Snowflakes

Serving Size: 36

2 cups all-purpose flour
1 cup unsweetened shredded coconut
1/2 cup maltitol
1 cup soft butter
1/4 cup milk
1 egg, well beaten
2 tsps vanilla extract

Preheat oven to 350°F. Combine all ingredients in a mixer bowl and mix until all ingredients are well combined, about 2-3 minutes. Drop by teaspoonfuls onto ungreased cookie sheets and bake for about 14 minutes, or until the edges are light brown. Remove from pan immediately.

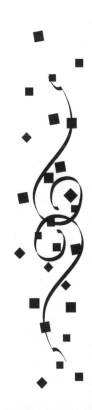

Coffee Crispies

Serving Size: 36

1 3/4 cups all-purpose flour
1/4 tsp salt
1/4 tsp baking soda
1/4 tsp baking powder
1 tbsp instant coffee powder
1/2 cup soft margarine
1/4 cup shortening
1/2 cup brown sugar replacement
1/2 cup maltitol
1 tsp vanilla extract
1 egg yolk

Preheat oven to 375°F. Stir together first 5 ingredients, set aside. Combine margarine and shortening and beat until fluffy. Add brown sugar replacement and beat well. Gradually add maltitol and beat well. Add vanilla and egg yolk and beat well. Add flour mixture and mix until no flour particles are visible. Shape dough into 1 inch balls and place on an ungreased cookie sheet 2 inches apart from each other. Flatten the cookies to a thickness of 1/4 inch with the bottom of a glass that has been dipped in water. Bake for about 10 minutes or until the cookies are golden brown. Allow cookies to sit on cookie sheet for 2 minutes before removing to cool completely on a rack.

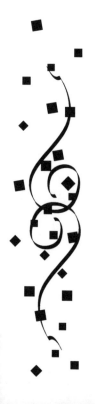

Cream Cheese Cookies

Serving Size: 48

1/2 cup unsalted butter at room temperature
3 ounces cream cheese at room temperature
2 cups maltitol
2 eggs
1 tsp vanilla extract
 grated peel of 1 lemon
4 cups all-purpose flour
1 tsp baking powder
1/2 tsp salt
1/2 cup apricot all-fruit preserves

Cream butter and cream cheese until light and fluffy. Add maltitol gradually, then eggs, one at a time, beating well after each addition. Stir in vanilla and lemon peel. Sift together flour, baking powder, and salt. Stir into buttercream cheese mixture.

Roll dough into a log about 18 inches long. Place on a 20-inch-long sheet of aluminum foil, roll up, and seal ends. Chill 2 hours.

To bake, preheat oven to 350°F. Slice dough into 3/8-inch-thick rounds and place on baking sheets that have been lightly sprayed with nonstick cooking spray. Spoon 1/2 teaspoon jam in center of each cookie. Bake until firm on top and golden brown on underside (8 to 10 minutes). Remove from baking sheet to a cooling rack.

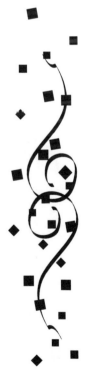

Double Chocolate Oatmeal Cookies

Serving Size: 96

1 1/4 cups all-purpose flour
1/3 cup unsweetened cocoa powder
1/2 tsp baking soda
1/2 tsp salt
1 cup soft margarine
1 cup maltitol
1/2 cup brown sugar replacement
1 egg
1/2 tsp vanilla extract
1/4 cup water
3 cups quick-cooking oats
12 ounces malt sweetened chocolate chips

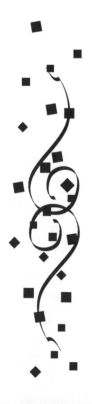

Preheat oven to 350°F. Sift together flour, cocoa, baking soda and salt, set aside. Combine brown sugar replacement and margarine and whip until very fluffy. Gradually add maltitol while mixing. Beat in egg and vanilla. Add flour mixture alternately with the water, mixing until smooth. Stir in oats, mix well. Stir in chocolate chips. Drop by teaspoonfuls onto ungreased cookie sheets about 1 1/2 inches apart from each other and bake for about 10 minutes or until lightly browned. Allow cookies to sit on cookie sheets for 3 minutes before removing to wire racks to cool completely.

Dutch Almond Cookies

Serving Size: 36

1 1/3 cups all-purpose flour
1/2 tsp baking powder
3/4 cup soft butter
1/2 cup brown sugar replacement
1/2 cup maltitol
1/2 tsp almond extract
2 tbsps water
1 cup sliced almonds (approximate amount)

Preheat oven to 325°F. Stir together flour and baking powder, set aside. Combine butter and brown sugar replacement and whip until very fluffy, then gradually add maltitol, mixing well. Mix in almond extract. Add flour mixture to butter mixture alternately with water, blending smooth after each addition. Spread almonds onto a plate and drop cookie dough by teaspoonfuls onto almonds. Roll each cookie to coat it well. Place cookies 1 inch apart onto ungreased cookie sheets. Bake 15-20 minutes or until lightly browned. Let cookies sit on cookie sheet 2 minutes before removing to racks to cool completely.

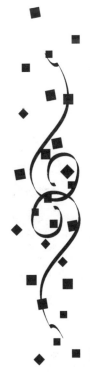

Gingerbread Cookies

Serving Size: 48

1/2 cup soft butter
2 1/2 cups all-purpose flour
1/2 cup maltitol
1 egg
1/4 cup brown sugar replacement
2 tsps baking powder
1 tsp ground ginger
1/2 tsp cinnamon
1/2 tsp allspice

Preheat oven to 375°F and spray cookie sheet(s) with nonstick cooking spray. Whip butter until light and fluffy, about 2-3 minutes. While still mixing, gradually add maltitol, then egg, mixing until well combined. Sift remaining ingredients together and add to the butter mixture, stirring until all the ingredients are combined. Cover dough and refrigerate for a few hours so it will be easier to handle.

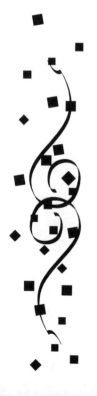

Cut dough in half and roll out one half of it at a time about 1/8 inch thick, then cut into your favorite shapes with a 2 inch cookie cutter. Place cookies about 1 inch apart on prepared cookie sheet and bake 5-6 minutes. Cool one minute on the cookie sheet, then transfer them to a rack to finish cooling.

Notes: Use as little flour as possible while rolling out to keep cookies tender.

Hazelnut Sandy Cookies

Serving Size: 36

8 tbsps unsalted butter, softened
1/4 cup maltitol
1 dash salt
1 egg yolk
1/2 tsp vanilla extract
1 cup all-purpose flour plus 2 tbsps
1/2 cup hazelnuts, chopped

Preheat oven to 325°F and lightly spray cookie sheet(s) with nonstick cooking spray, set aside. Whip butter until fluffy and white, then while mixing, gradually add maltitol, then salt, then egg yolk, then vanilla, beating well after each addition. Turn mixer to low and mix in flour and hazelnuts. Shape the dough into a cylinder about 8 inch long, then wrap it in a piece of plastic wrap, chill until it is very firm. Remove the plastic and slice the dough into 1/4 inch pieces, and set them on the baking sheets a little apart from each other. Bake the cookies about 15 minutes, or until they are a light golden color. Let the cookies cool 10 minutes on the pan then transfer them to finish cooking on a rack.

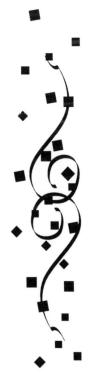

Hermits

Serving Size: 60

1 1/4 cups seedless raisins
2 1/2 cups all-purpose flour
1/2 tsp baking soda
1 tsp cream of tartar
1/2 tsp ground cloves
1/2 tsp cinnamon
1/2 tsp allspice
1/2 tsp ginger
1/2 tsp ground nutmeg
1/2 cup butter
1 cup maltitol
1/4 cup skim milk

Chop raisins finely in food processor with 1/4 cup flour. Sift 2 cups flour with soda, cream of tartar, and spices. Cream butter with maltitol. Add dry ingredients alternately with milk until well blended. Stir in raisins and enough additional flour, up to 3/4 cup, to make a stiff dough. Shape into two logs, about 1-1/2 inch diameter. Chill overnight. When ready to make, slice 1/4 inch thin and bake at 375°F until done, about 15-20 minutes

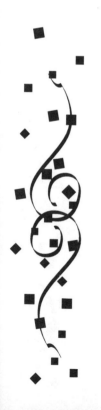

Honey Almond Treats

Serving Size: 48

1 1/2 cups all-purpose flour
1 tsp baking soda
1/2 cup soft butter
1/2 cup shortening
1 cup maltitol, honey flavored
1/2 tsp vanilla extract
1/4 tsp almond extract
1 cup sliced almonds

Stir together flour and baking soda, set aside. Whip butter and
shortening together until it is light and fluffy, then gradually
add maltitol. Add extracts. Add flour mixture, combine well.
Stir in almonds by hand. Divide dough in half and shape each
into a log that is 2 inches across. Wrap the logs in plastic wrap
and refrigerate until firm, at least 2 hours. Preheat oven to
350°F and spray cookie sheet(s) with nonstick cooking spray.
Slice cookies 1/4 inch thin and arrange on cookie sheet 1 1/2
inches apart. Bake cookies about 10 minutes, or until golden
brown. Allow cookies to sit on cookie sheet for 2 minutes
before removing to a rack to cool completely.

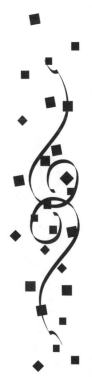

Lemon Chews

Serving Size: 48

2 1/2 cups all-purpose flour
1 1/4 cups maltitol
3/4 cup unsweetened shredded coconut
1 cup soft butter
2 eggs, well beaten
1 1/2 tsps cream of tartar
1 tsp baking soda
1 tbsp fresh lemon juice
1 tsp grated lemon zest

Preheat oven to 400°F. Combine all ingredients in a large
mixer bowl and mix until all ingredients are combined and no
traces of flour are left. Drop by teaspoonfuls onto ungreased
cookie sheets and bake about 8-10 minutes, or until they are
lightly browned. Remove from pan immediately.

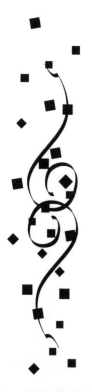

Lemon Pecan Cookies

Serving Size: 48

2 3/4 cups all-purpose flour
1 1/2 cups maltitol
3/4 cup soft butter
2 eggs, well beaten
1 tsp baking soda
1/2 tsp cream of tartar
 dash salt
2 tbsps fresh lemon juice
1 tbsp grated lemon zest
1 tsp vanilla extract
1 cup chopped pecans

Preheat oven to 400°F. Combine all ingredients, except pecans, and mix until well blended, about 3 minutes. Add pecans and mix just until they are evenly dispersed. Shape teaspoonfuls into 1 inch balls and place on an ungreased cookie sheet 2 inches apart from each other. Bake for about 8 minutes, or until edges begin to brown. Remove form cookie sheet immediately.

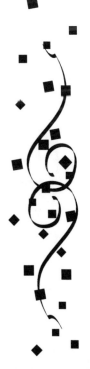

Lemon Poppyseed Cookies

Serving Size: 50

1 cup butter, softened
1 cup maltitol
1 egg
2 tsps poppy seeds
1 tsp lemon extract
2 cups all-purpose flour

Preheat oven to 375°F. Whip butter until light and fluffy then gradually add maltitol while mixing. Add egg and mix well. Add poppy seeds and extract and mix well. Sift flour over dough and mix until no traces of flour are left. Roll dough into a cylinder with a 2 inch diameter and wrap with plastic wrap. Refrigerate one hour. Cut dough with a sharp knife into 1/4 inch slices and place the slices on an ungreased cookie sheet. Bake 8-10 minutes or until the edges are firm. Cool on sheet for 11 minute, then transfer to a wire rack to cool completely.

Notes: This recipe is also excellent using orange extract instead of lemon.

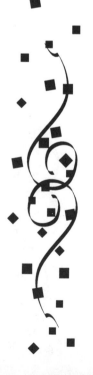

Linzer Cookies

Serving Size: 24

3/4 cup butter, softened
1/2 cup maltitol
1 egg
1/2 tsp lemon zest, grated
1 dash salt
1/2 tsp cinnamon
2 cups all-purpose flour
1 cup hazelnuts, ground very fine
1/4 cup raspberry jam, no sugar added

Preheat oven to 350°F. Whip butter until light and slowly add maltitol, then egg, then lemon zest, salt and cinnamon. Add in flour and ground nuts just until combined. Take 1 tablespoon of the mixture, roll it into a ball, then press it out into a flat circle, 1/4 inch thick. Repeat this until all batter is used. Place raw cookies on a cookie sheet that has been lightly sprayed with nonstick cooking spray and top each one with 1/2 teaspoon of fruit spread. Bake at for about 20 minutes, or until the outer edge of the cookie is firm. Cool 5 minutes on cookie sheet before removing them to cool completely.

Notes: Ground almonds can be substituted for the hazelnuts, if you like.

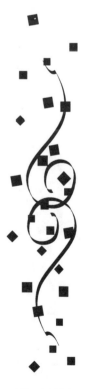

Low-Fat Delicate Lemon Cake Cookies

Serving Size: 78

1 cup cake flour, sifted
1 1/4 tsps baking powder
 dash nutmeg
2 eggs at room temperature
1/2 cup maltitol
2 tsps grated lemon zest
2 tsps fresh lemon juice

Preheat oven to 400°F and generously spray cookie sheet(s) with nonstick cooking spray, set aside. Sift together flour, baking powder, and nutmeg, set aside. Whip eggs until thick, then gradually add maltitol until mixture is thick and very pale. Add in lemon zest and juice. Gradually add flour mixture and mix until just blended. Drop by teaspoons onto prepared cookie sheet and bake about 5 minutes or until edges are light brown. Remove from cookie sheet immediately.

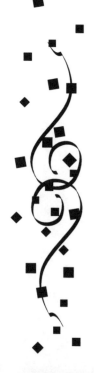

Luscious Lemon Cookies

Serving Size: 72

4 cups all-purpose flour
1 tsp baking powder
1/2 tsp baking soda
1/2 tsp salt
1 cup butter, softened
1 1/2 cups maltitol
1 large egg
1/2 cup sour cream
2 tsps lemon extract
2 tbsps lemon peel, grated
3 tbsps lemon juice

Sift flour with baking powder, baking soda and salt. In large bowl of electric mixer, beat butter, maltitol and egg at medium speed until light and fluffy. At low speed, beat in sour cream, lemon extract and grated lemon peel until smooth. Gradually add flour mixture, beating until well combined. Form dough into a ball, wrap in foil and refrigerate overnight. Divide dough into 4 parts. Refrigerate until ready to roll out. On floured surface roll dough, one part at a time, 1/4-inch thick. Using a 2 to 3-inch cookie cutter or glass, cut out cookies. Use a spatula to carefully pick up and place cookies on a lightly greased cookie sheet 2 inches apart. Lightly brush cookies with lemon juice. Bake in preheated 375°F oven for 10-12 minutes until golden brown. Do not overcook. Remove cookies to wire rack to cool completely. Complete baking using one part cookie dough at a time, greasing the pan each time.

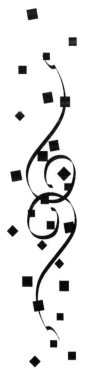

Macadamia Nut Cookies

Serving Size: 60

1 cup all-purpose flour
1/4 tsp baking soda
1/2 cup soft butter
1/2 cup brown sugar replacement
3/4 cup maltitol
1 egg, well beaten
1 tsp vanilla extract
1 cup chopped macadamia nuts

Preheat oven to 375°F and lightly spray cookie sheet(s) with nonstick cooking spray, set aside. Combine flour and baking soda, set aside. Combine brown sugar substitute and butter and whip until butter is very fluffy. Gradually add maltitol while mixing, then add egg and vanilla. Add flour to butter mixture and mix until well combined, about 2 minutes. Stir in macadamia nuts by hand. Drop by teaspoonfuls onto prepared cookie sheet and bake about 8 minutes, or until cookies are golden brown. Let cookies sit on cookie sheet 2 minutes before removing them to a wire rack to cool completely.

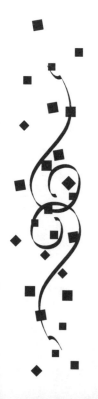

Madeleines

Serving Size: 15

1/2 cup unsalted butter
2 eggs
1/2 cup maltitol
1 tsp grated lemon zest
1/4 tsp lemon juice
1/4 tsp vanilla extract
1/8 tsp baking powder
3/4 cup sifted cake flour

Place the butter in a saucepan over medium heat and melt the butter, cooking it just until the milk solids turn a golden brown color, set aside to cool. Place a medium bowl over a pot of simmering water and place in it the eggs and maltitol. Whisk the mixture until it is body temperature, then remove from the heat. Add the lemon zest, juice and vanilla to it. Sift the cake flour and baking powder into the mixture, combine well. Stir in the melted and cooled butter. Cover bowl with plastic wrap and let the mixture rest for 1 hour. Preheat oven to 450°F. Brush the insides of madeleine pans with a thin layer of butter and dust them lightly with flour. Invert the pan and rap it on the counter to remove any excess flour. Spoon the batter into the shells, filling them 3/4 full. Bake for about 10-12 minutes (for 3 inch madeleines) or until they spring back when lightly touched. Invert pan onto rack to cool madeleines. Best served warm.

Notes: Madeleines are delicate little cookies that are baked in a special pan that has rows of indentations that look like shells. They are succulent treats, great for teatime.

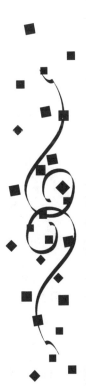

Meringue Hearts

Serving Size: 6

3 egg whites
1 tsp vanilla extract
1/4 tsp cream of tartar
1 dash salt
1 cup maltitol
1 pint strawberries, sliced

Cut a heart pattern from a 4-1/2 inch square of paper. Cover baking sheet with brown paper. (You can bake on the brown paper so make sure it is clean.) Grocery store bags without writing on them are okay. Draw 6 hearts on the brown paper using your pattern as a guide. Beat egg whites with vanilla, cream of tartar and salt until frothy. Add maltitol, a little at a time, and continue beating until stiff peaks form. Spread meringue over the heart shapes, 1/4 inch thick. Make into the heart shape using a spoon to push and form into correct shape. Pipe rim 3/4 inch high with pastry tube. Bake in preheated 275°F oven for 1 hour. Turn off oven and let meringues dry in oven for 1 more hour. DO NOT open oven door during this time. Fill the cooled meringues with strawberries. Decorate with mint leaves if desired.

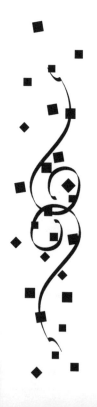

Minty Chocolate Cookies

Serving Size: 96

2 cups maltitol
1 cup unsweetened cocoa powder, sifted
1 cup soft butter
1 cup buttermilk or sour milk
1 cup water
2 eggs, well beaten
2 tsps baking soda
1 tsp baking powder
1/2 tsp salt
2 tsps mint extract
4 cups all-purpose flour

Preheat oven to 400°F and spray cookie sheet(s) with nonstick cooking spray, set aside. Combine all ingredients, except flour, and mix until well combined, about 3 minutes. Add flour and mix until well combined, about 3 minutes more. Drop teaspoonfuls of dough onto prepared cookie sheet and bake about 8 minutes, or until top of cookie springs back when touched lightly. Remove from cookie sheet immediately.

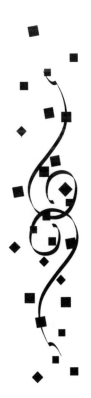

Oatmeal Cookies

Serving Size: 72

1 cup butter, softened
2 cups all-purpose flour
1 tsp cinnamon
1 tsp baking soda
1 tsp double-acting baking powder
1/2 cup brown sugar replacement
1 1/2 cups maltitol
2 eggs, beaten slightly
3 cups rolled oats
1/2 cup seedless raisins

Preheat oven to 350°F and spray cookie sheet(s) with nonstick cooking spray. Melt butter and cool to room temperature. Sift flour, cinnamon, baking soda, and baking powder together. Add brown sugar replacement and maltitol to butter and stir well. Add eggs, sifted dry ingredients, oats, and raisins. Drop by spoonfuls onto cookie sheets. Bake for 10 minutes.

Notes: If you don't care for raisins, add any dried fruit instead.

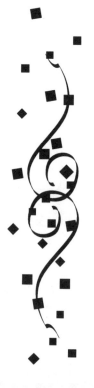

Oatmeal Sandwich Cookies

Serving Size: 50

Cookie:
1 cup butter, melted
1 1/3 cups maltitol
1/3 cup skim milk
1 1/3 cups rolled oats
1 1/2 cups all-purpose flour
1 tsp baking powder
1 tsp vanilla extract
Filling:
1 tbsp all-purpose flour
1/4 cup maltitol
2/3 cup skim milk
2 egg yolks
1/2 cup soft butter

Preheat oven to 350°F and spray cookie sheet(s) with nonstick cooking spray. Combine all cookie ingredients and mix thoroughly. Drop by teaspoonfuls onto prepared cookie sheets. Bake for 10-12 minutes or until golden brown. Cool 2 minutes, then remove carefully from cookie sheets to wire rack. Combine 1 tablespoon flour and 1 tablespoon maltitol in saucepan over low heat. Gradually add 2/3 cup milk and 2 egg yolks. Mix well. Cook over low heat, stirring constantly, until mixture is thick. Cool to room temperature. Cream butter then add 1/4 cup maltitol, creaming well. Gradually add egg mixture, beating well after each addition. To assemble cookies, spoon a little of the filling on the flat side of one cookie and press another cookie on top of the filling.

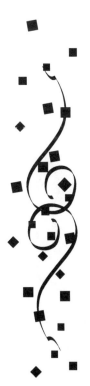

Orange and Honey Spice Cookies

Serving Size: 36

2 cups all-purpose flour
1 cup maltitol, honey flavored
3/4 cup soft butter
1 egg, well beaten
1/2 tsp baking soda
1/2 tsp nutmeg
1/4 tsp allspice
1/2 tsp orange extract

Preheat oven to 375°F. Combine all ingredients and mix well, about 3 minutes. Drop by teaspoonfuls onto ungreased cookie sheets about 2 inches apart from each other. Bake for about 8 minutes, or until the edges are light brown. Remove from cookie sheet immediately.

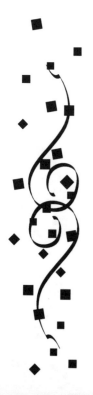

Orange-Coconut Drops

Serving Size: 60

1 3/4 cups maltitol
1 cup soft butter
3 eggs, well beaten
1 tsp baking powder
1/4 tsp salt
1 tsp vanilla extract
1 tsp orange extract
3 1/2 cups all-purpose flour
1/2 cup unsweetened shredded coconut

Preheat oven to 350°F and spray cookie sheet(s) with nonstick cooking spray, set aside. Combine maltitol, butter, and eggs and mix until very well combined. Add baking powder, salt and extracts. Combine flour and coconut and add to mixture while mixer is on, stirring until well mixed. Drop teaspoonfuls of dough onto prepared cookie sheets and bake for about 10 minutes, or until the edges are browned.

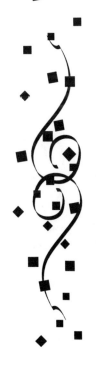

Peanut Butter Cookies

Serving Size: 60

2 cups all-purpose flour
3/4 tsp baking soda
1/2 tsp double-acting baking powder
1/4 tsp salt
1/2 cup shortening
1 cup peanut butter
1/2 cup brown sugar replacement
1/2 cup maltitol
1 egg

Preheat oven to 375°F and spray cookie sheet(s) with nonstick cooking spray. Sift flour, baking soda, baking powder, and salt together. Cream butter and peanut butter together. Gradually beat in brown sugar replacement and maltitol syrup. Add egg and beat until fluffy. Stir in dry ingredients. Roll dough, a teaspoonful at a time, into balls; place 3 inches apart on cookie sheets; flatten with fork. Bake for 12 minutes, or until golden brown. Let cookies cool on pan 5 minutes before removing them to a rack to cool completely.

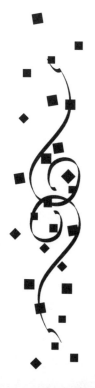

Pecan Sandies

Serving Size: 144

2 cups butter
1 cup maltitol
5 cups all-purpose flour
2 tsps vanilla extract
2 cups pecans, chopped

Preheat oven to 325°F. In a mixing bowl, cream the butter and maltitol, add flour, vanilla and pecans. Mix well. Roll dough into 1-inch balls and place on ungreased cookie sheets. Bake for 17-20 minutes or until lightly browned. Allow cookies to cool 5 minutes on pan before removing to a rack to finish cooling.

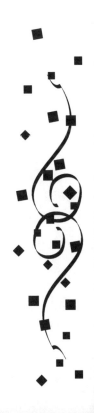

Pina Colada Cookies

Serving Size: 36

1/2 cup maltitol
1/2 cup soft butter
2 eggs
1/3 cup pineapple all-fruit preserves, no sugar added
1/2 tsp baking powder
1/4 tsp salt
1 tsp rum extract
1 3/4 cups all-purpose flour
1/3 cup unsweetened shredded coconut

Preheat oven to 350°F and spray cookie sheet(s) with nonstick cooking spray, set aside. Combine maltitol, butter, preserves, baking powder, salt, and rum extract and beat until well combined. Combine flour and coconut and add to butter mixture, stirring until well combined, about 3 minutes. Drop by teaspoonfuls onto prepared cookie sheet 2 inches apart from each other. Bake about 10 minutes, or until edges are light brown. Remove from cookie sheet immediately.

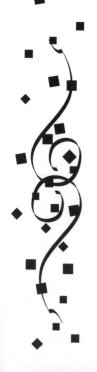

Pine Nut Crescents

Serving Size: 30

2 cups all-purpose flour
1/4 tsp nutmeg
2/3 cup soft butter
1/3 cup brown sugar replacement
1/4 cup maltitol
2 egg yolks
1 tbsp grated orange zest
3/4 cup pine nuts (pignolia)

Preheat oven to 350°F and spray cookie sheet(s) with nonstick cooking spray, set aside. Combine flour and nutmeg, set aside. Combine butter and brown sugar replacement and whip until very fluffy. Gradually add maltitol, beat well. Add egg yolks, one at a time, beating well after each addition. Blend in orange zest. Add flour mixture to the butter mixture and mix until thoroughly combined. Scoop out dough, one tablespoon at a time, and shape each one into a 3 inch long crescent. Take each crescent and press it into the pine nuts, covering the top completely. Bake the cookies about 10 minutes or until they are golden. Allow them to cool on the baking sheet for 2 minutes before removing them to a rack to cool completely.

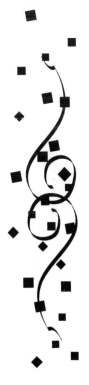

Purist Peanut Butter Cookies

Serving Size: 24

1 cup peanut butter, no sugar added
2/3 cup maltitol
1 egg

Preheat oven to 350°F and spray cookie sheet with nonstick cooking spray. In a medium bowl combine peanut butter, maltitol, and egg - blend well. Form dough into 1-inch balls. Place 1-1/2 to 2 inches apart on cookie sheet. Using a fork, press a crisscross pattern into dough. Bake 12 to 15 minutes, or until lightly browned. Cool on wire rack.

Raisin Cookies

Serving Size: 84

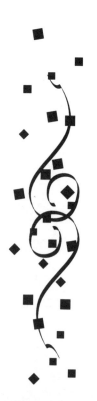

3 1/2 cups all-purpose flour
1/2 cup brown sugar replacement
3/4 cup maltitol
1 cup soft butter
1 cup milk
2 eggs, well beaten
2 tsps baking powder
1/4 tsp salt
1 tsp vanilla extract
1 cup raisins

Preheat oven to 375°F and spray cookie sheet(s) with nonstick cooking spray, set aside. Combine all ingredients, except raisins, and mix well, about 3 minutes. Add raisins and mix until raisins are evenly dispersed. Drop dough by teaspoonfuls onto prepared cookie sheet 2 inches apart from each other. Bake for about 10 minutes, or until edges begin to brown. Remove from cookie sheet immediately.

Ranger Cookies

Serving Size: 42

1 cup all-purpose flour
1/2 tsp baking soda
1/4 tsp baking powder
 dash salt
1/2 cup soft butter
1/2 cup brown sugar replacement
1/2 cup maltitol
1 egg
1 tsp vanilla extract
1 cup quick-cooking oats
1 cup crispy rice cereal
1/2 cup unsweetened shredded coconut

Preheat oven to 375°F and lightly spray cookie sheet(s) with nonstick cooking spray, set aside. Sift together first 4 ingredients, set aside. Combine butter and brown sugar replacement and whip until very fluffy. Gradually add maltitol, egg and vanilla, mix well. Add flour mixture and mix for about 2 minutes, or until well combined. By hand, stir in oats, cereal and coconut. Drop by teaspoonfuls onto prepared cookie sheet and bake for about 10 minutes or until the cookies are golden brown. Remove from cookie sheets immediately.

Notes: This recipe is a timeless classic.

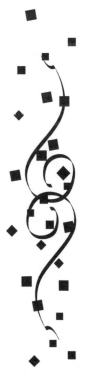

Sour Cream Coconut Crisps

Serving Size: 54

1 1/2 cups all-purpose flour
1/4 tsp baking soda
1/4 tsp baking powder
 dash salt
1 1/2 cups unsweetened shredded coconut
1/2 cup soft butter
1/2 cup maltitol
1/2 cup brown sugar replacement
2 tsps grated orange zest
1 egg yolk
1/4 cup sour cream

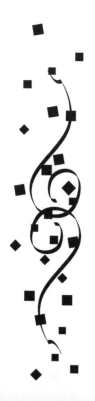

Combine first 5 ingredients, set aside. Whip the butter until it is light and fluffy, then add maltitol gradually, beating well. Add brown sugar replacement and beat well. Blend in orange zest. Add egg yolk and sour cream, beat until fluffy. Gradually beat in flour mixture, mix until thoroughly combined. Divide dough in half and shape each into a log 2 inches across. Wrap the logs in plastic wrap and refrigerate until firm, at least 2 hours. Preheat oven to 375°F and spray cookie sheet(s) with nonstick cooking spray. Slice cookies into 1/4 inch thick slices and arrange them on sheet 1 inch apart from each other. Bake for about 10 minutes, or until cookies are golden.

Spiced Honey Cookies

Serving Size: 24

3/4 cup unsalted butter, softened
1 1/4 cups maltitol, honey flavored
1 egg
2 cups flour
2 tsps baking powder
1 tsp ground cinnamon
3/4 tsp ground ginger
1/4 tsp ground cloves
1/4 tsp salt

Preheat oven to 375°F and spray cookie sheet(s) with nonstick cooking spray, set aside. In large bowl of electric mixer, cream butter and maltitol until light and fluffy. Mix in egg. Combine flour, baking soda, cinnamon, ginger, cloves, and salt. Add to butter mixture, mixing thoroughly. Form dough into small balls. Place 1-1/2 to 2 inches apart on cookie sheets. Bake 10 to 15 minutes. Remove to wire rack to cool.

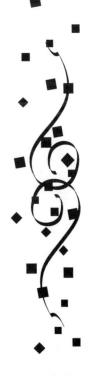

Spicy Date Cookies

Serving Size: 72

2 1/2 cups all-purpose flour
3/4 tsp baking soda
1/2 tsp salt
1 tsp ground cinnamon
1/4 tsp ground cloves
1/4 tsp ground allspice
1 cup butter, softened
1 cup maltitol
3 large eggs
1 tsp vanilla extract
8 ounces dates pitted, chopped
1 cup walnuts, chopped

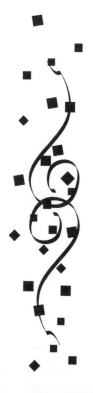

Preheat oven to 400°F and lightly spray cookie sheet(s) with nonstick cooking spray, set aside. Sift together the flour, baking soda, salt, and spices, set aside. Place softened butter into large mixer bowl. Add maltitol, eggs and vanilla, one at a time. Beat until smooth and fluffy using medium speed. Stir in flour mixture with a wooden spoon until well combined. Stir in dates and walnuts. Cover tightly and refrigerate for 1 hour or more. Drop by rounded teaspoonfuls, 2 inches apart, onto cookie sheets. Bake for 8-10 minutes or until lightly browned. Transfer to wire rack and cool completely.

Super Rich Chocolate Cookies

Serving Size: 54

1 cup almonds, ground
1 ounce unsweetened chocolate squares, chopped fine
1 cup soft butter
2/3 cup maltitol
1 tsp vanilla extract
1/4 tsp almond extract
1 1/4 cups all-purpose flour

Preheat oven to 275°F. Whip butter in a mixer until it is light and fluffy, then gradually add maltitol while mixing. Add both extracts and chopped chocolate. With mixer on low, gradually add flour and ground nuts, mix until well combined. Drop cookies by teaspoonfuls onto ungreased cookie sheets and bake for about 35 minutes, or until they are firm. Allow cookies to cool 5 minutes on cookie sheets before removing them to a rack to cool completely.

Notes: It is very important that the chocolate is cut into very small pieces, almost ground.

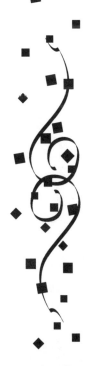

Tahini Cookies

Serving Size: 36

1 1/2 cups all-purpose flour
2 tsps baking powder
1/4 tsp ground cardamom
 dash salt
1/2 cup soft butter
1/2 cup tahini
1/2 cup maltitol
1/2 cup brown sugar replacement
1 egg yolk
 sesame seeds, optional

Preheat oven to 375°F. Combine first 4 ingredients, set aside. Combine butter and tahini and beat until fluffy. Add maltitol and brown sugar replacement and beat well. Add vanilla and egg yolk, beating until fluffy. Gradually add flour mixture, beating until well combined. Shape dough into 1 inch balls and place them on an ungreased cookie sheet about 1 1/2 inches apart from each other. Press them down slightly with your fingers. If desired, sprinkle the cookies with sesame seeds. Bake for about 10 minutes or until the cookies are lightly browned.

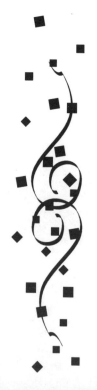

Thumbprint Cookies

Serving Size: 36

2 cups all-purpose flour
1/4 cup brown sugar replacement
1/4 cup maltitol
1 cup soft butter
2 egg yolks
 dash salt
1/2 tsp vanilla extract
 all-fruit preserves, no sugar added

Preheat oven to 350°F and spray cookie sheet(s) with nonstick
cooking spray, set aside. Combine all ingredients, except
preserves, and mix for about 2 minutes or until a nice dough
is formed. Scoop out dough by teaspoonfuls and shape them
into little balls. Place the balls onto the prepared cookie sheet
and press into the middle of them with your thumb, leaving a
small indention. Fill the indentions with a teaspoon or so of
preserves. Bake for about 15 minutes, or until cookies are light
brown and firm.

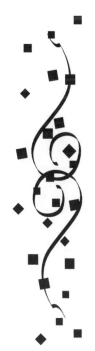

Vanilla Bean Butter Cookies

Serving Size: 30

3/4 cup maltitol
1 cup soft butter
2 egg yolks
1 vanilla bean
2 cups all-purpose flour
1/8 tsp salt
 whole almonds, optional

Preheat oven to 350°F. Combine maltitol, butter and egg yolks and mix until combined. Split the vanilla bean down the middle and use a small knife to scrape out the vanilla inside. Scrape the vanilla into the butter mixture, discard the bean. Mix again until the vanilla looks evenly dispersed. Scrape the bowl down and add the flour and salt and mix until no particles of flour can be seen. Shape teaspoonfuls of dough into 1 inch balls and place them on an ungreased cookie sheet, 2 inches apart from each other. Press the balls out to 1/4 inch thickness with the bottom of a glass dipped in water. If desired, place an almond in the center of each cookie. Bake for about 10 minutes, or until the edges are lightly browned. Cool 1 minute on the pan before removing to a rack to cool completely.

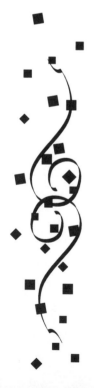

Yummy Pumpkin Cookies

Serving Size: 60

1 1/2 cups all-purpose flour
1/2 tsp baking powder
1 1/2 tsps pumpkin pie spice
1/4 tsp baking soda
1/4 tsp salt
1/2 cup soft butter
1/2 cup brown sugar replacement
2/3 cup maltitol
1 egg
1/2 tsp vanilla extract
1 cup pumpkin puree
1/2 cup raisins, soaked in hot water
1/2 cup chopped nuts, optional

Preheat oven to 350°F and spray cookie sheet(s) with nonstick cooking spray, set aside. Sift together first 5 ingredients, set aside. Combine butter and brown sugar replacement and whip until fluffy, then gradually add maltitol while mixing. Add egg and vanilla, mix well. Add flour mixture alternately with pumpkin, mixing until all ingredients are well blended, about 2 minutes. Remove raisins form hot water and squeeze out any excess water and add them to the dough. Add nuts, if desired. Drop by teaspoonfuls onto prepared cookie sheet and bake for about 20 minutes, or until top feels firm when touched lightly.

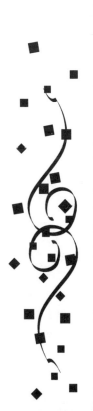

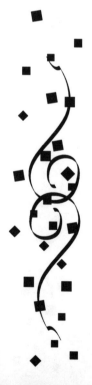

sweets *with a*
foreign
flair

Apple Strudel

Serving Size: 12

4 large Granny Smith apples
1/2 cup brown sugar replacement
1 tsp cinnamon
1/4 tsp cardamom
1/4 cup almond slivers
1/2 cup butter, melted
4 sheets phyllo dough
2 tbsps bread crumbs

Preheat oven to 400°F and spray a baking sheet with nonstick cooking spray. Peel, core, and finely chop apples. Mix with brown sugar replacement, spices, nuts, and 2 tablespoons melted butter. Unwrap phyllo dough and keep between two dampened towels. Place one sheet of dough on another damp towel. Brush with melted butter and sprinkle with bread crumbs. Place second sheet of phyllo on top of first, brush with butter, and sprinkle with crumbs. Repeat with remaining sheets of phyllo. Spread apple filling, about two inches in, along one long side of dough, to within two inches of each edge. Filling should be spread about three inches wide. Fold long side over once to cover filling, then fold in edges. Continue to roll lengthwise, like a jelly roll, using towel to help. Brush each roll with butter, and place, seam side down, on baking sheet. Bake about 20-25 minutes, until golden. Remove from oven and score top into 1-1/2 inch slices with a sharp knife. Cool and cut into slices.

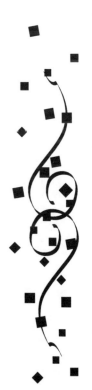

Babas au Rhum

Serving Size: 24

1 package dry yeast
1 1/2 cups all-purpose flour
4 large eggs
1/4 cup maltitol
1/8 tsp salt
1/2 cup margarine, softened
1 cup maltitol
1/2 cup rum

Place 1/2 cup lukewarm water in a mixing bowl; sprinkle yeast over water. Let stand 5 minutes to soften. Add 1/2 cup flour and beat well with electric mixer. Beat in the eggs one at a time, then the salt, maltitol, and remaining 1 cup flour. Cover and let rise until doubled, about 45 minutes. Beat in the softened margarine a tablespoon at a time. Spray cupcake tins or pans made especially for babas with nonstick cooking spray. Put 1 tablespoon of batter in each tin. Cover and let stand for 10 minutes. Bake in preheated 400°F oven until browned. Time will depend on size of pan you are using. Cool babas.

To make the sauce, boil 1 cup water with maltitol for 10 minutes. Cool to lukewarm and add 1/2 rum. Dip cooled cakes in this mixture and pour more sauce around them. Babas are traditionally very moist with the syrup.

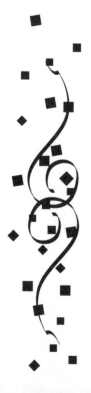

Quick Hints
Working with Phyllo
Spraying phyllo sheets with olive oil or melted butter from a spritzer bottle is a fast, easy way to apply the fat in a very thin layer.

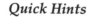

Baklava

Serving Size: 36

2 1/2 cups maltitol, honey flavored
1/2 cup hot water
1 tbsp lemon juice
1 pound walnuts, chopped
1/4 cup brown sugar replacement
1/2 tsp cinnamon
1/8 tsp nutmeg
1 pound phyllo dough
1 cup butter, melted

To prepare syrup, combine maltitol, water and lemon juice, set aside. Preheat oven to 325°F and spray a 13X9X2 inch baking pan generously with nonstick cooking spray, set aside. Mix walnuts, 1/4 cup brown sugar replacement, and spices; set aside. Keep phyllo pastry covered with a damp towel while working with individual sheets. Layer sheets in baking pan, one at a time, brushing each layer with melted butter (or if you have a spray bottle, spray the butter over the sheets). After layering six or so, begin alternating layers of phyllo pastry with nut mixture. Brush one layer with butter and sprinkle the next with 1/2 cup nut mixture. Continue to alternate buttered layers and nut-covered layers until all but ten of the sheets have been used. Layer the last ten sheets as you did the bottom six, brushing each with butter. Bake for 1-1/2 hours. Remove from oven and let cool for five minutes. Score pastry into diamond shapes about 1-1/2 inch X 2 inch. Pour cold syrup over hot pastry. Allow to cool to room temperature before cutting and removing from pan.

Notes: If you prefer a nut other than walnuts, feel free to use another. Nuts that are particularly good in baklava are: almonds, pecans, and pistachios.

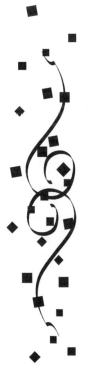

Biscotti

Serving Size: 18

4 cups flour
1 1/2 cups maltitol
1/2 tsp salt
2 tsps baking powder
2/3 cup butter, cold
4 whole eggs
1 tsp vanilla extract
1 tsp almond extract
1 tbsp anise seed
1 cup almonds, ground

Sift together flour, salt, and baking powder. Cut butter into mixture. Beat eggs slightly and beat in maltitol, vanilla and almond extracts. Quickly stir egg mixture, anise seed, and almonds into dry ingredients. Turn out on a floured board and knead until dough is no longer sticky. Divide dough into 6-8 pieces. Roll with hands into long rolls. Place rolls on greased baking pans and flatten slightly with hands. Bake at 325°F for 25-30 minutes. Slice each roll diagonally into 3/4 inch pieces. Return to baking pan, cut side up, and bake at 375°F for 5 minutes. Turn biscotti over and bake 5 minutes more.

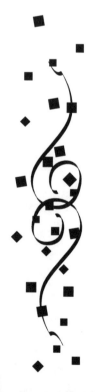

Blueberry Streusel

Serving Size: 12

1/2 cup butter
1/2 cup maltitol
1 egg
2 cups all-purpose flour
2 tsps double-acting baking powder
1/2 tsp baking soda
1/4 tsp salt
1/2 cup lowfat buttermilk
2 cups fresh blueberries
1/4 cup butter cold
1/2 cup flour
1 tsp cinnamon
1/2 tsp ground nutmeg
1/2 cup brown sugar replacement

Preheat oven to 350°F and spray a 13X9X2 inch baking pan with nonstick cooking spray. Cream maltitol and butter. Beat in egg. Sift dry ingredients together and add, alternately with buttermilk, to butter mixture. Pour into pan. Top with blueberries. Mix brown sugar replacement, flour, and spices. Cut butter into tablespoons and blend into dry ingredients with a pastry blender. Mixture should be crumbly. Sprinkle over blueberries. Bake for 35 minutes. Serve warm.

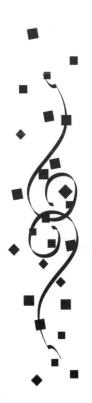

Chocolate Almond Biscotti

Serving Size: 30

1/2 cup soft butter
1 cup maltitol
2 large eggs
1 1/2 tbsps coffee liqueur
2 1/4 cups all-purpose flour
1 1/2 tsps baking powder
1/4 tsp salt
1 1/2 tbsps unsweetened cocoa powder, sifted
1 cup whole almonds

Preheat oven to 350°F and lightly spray a cookie sheet with nonstick cooking spray, set aside. Combine butter and maltitol and whip until very light, add eggs, one at a time, beating well after each addition. Add coffee liqueur, beat well. Sift together flour, baking powder, salt and cocoa powder then add it to the butter mixture, mix well. Stir in almonds. Divide dough in half and shape each into a 9X2 inch log on the cookie sheet. Press down slightly on the tops of the logs to flatten them a little. Bake cookies for about 30 minutes, or until they are firm. Set aside to cool enough so that they can be handled. Cut each log diagonally across into 1/2 inch thick slices and place the slices on an ungreased cookie sheet. Bake the cookies for about 5 minutes, turn them over and cook for 5 more minutes, or until the cookies are dry.

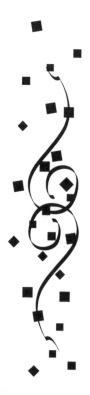

Quick Hints
Shapely Biscotti
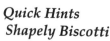
Turn the dough into a greased, metal ice cube tray, without the cube insert, and bake it right in the tray! This prevents overhandling and comes out in a neat, easy-to-slice loaf. After slicing the loaf, toast the biscotti on a cookie sheet.

Coeurs a la Creme (Cream Cheese Hearts)

Serving Size: 4

cheesecloth, rinsed
8 ounces lowfat cream cheese, softened
1 cup heavy cream
1 tsp Equal® sweetener
1/2 tsp vanilla extract
2 egg whites at room temperature
2 cups fresh raspberries or strawberries

Combine cream cheese, cream, Equal and vanilla and mix until very soft. Whip the egg whites to stiff peaks and fold them into the cheese mixture. Line coeurs a la creme molds with a few layers of cheesecloth and spoon the mixture into them, smoothing the tops. Fold the remaining cheesecloth over the tops of the molds to enclose it completely. Place the molds on a flat dish and refrigerate them overnight (you may want to cover the molds on the plate with plastic wrap to prevent them from absorbing refrigerator odors). To serve, remove molds from the refrigerator and unwrap the tops. Place a dessert plate on top the mold and invert, them carefully remove the remaining cheesecloth. Surround dessert with berries and serve.

Notes: This recipe uses special heart shaped molds with holes on the bottom so it can drain, but any mold that can drain will do.

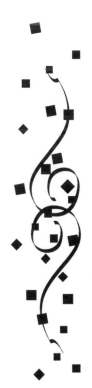

Creme Anglaise (Vanilla Sauce)

Serving Size: 10

1 cup milk
1 cup heavy cream
1/2 cup maltitol
1/2 vanilla bean
6 egg yolks

Place milk, cream, maltitol and vanilla bean in a heavy bottomed sauce pot, do not stir. Bring the mixture to a boil over medium heat. Whisk one cup of the hot mixture into the egg yolks. Add the egg yolk mixture to the boiling mixture all at once, stirring constantly. Remove pot from the heat immediately. Strain sauce if desired, remove vanilla bean and scrape out seeds from inside into the sauce. Discard the bean. This sauce can be served warm or cold.

Notes: The process of heating up egg yolks with some of a hot mixture before adding them to the mixture is called "tempering". It is done to slowly heat up the yolks so they do not curdle when they are added to a hot mixture.

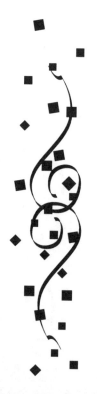

Creme Fraiche

Serving Size: 5

1/2 cup whipping cream, not ultra pasteurized
1 1/2 tsps buttermilk

Combine cream and buttermilk in a small jar. Cover jar and shake well to mix. Let mixture stand at room temperature 4 to 8 hours; it will thicken slightly and will thicken more when chilled. Store in the refrigerator.

Notes: Creme Fraiche is heavenly as an accompaniment to any fruit dish.

Crepes

Serving Size: 12

2 large eggs
2/3 cup milk
1 tbsp butter, melted
1/2 cup all-purpose flour
1/4 tsp salt
 vegetable oil

Beat eggs thoroughly. Blend in melted butter and milk. Stir in flour only until smooth. Lightly brush a 5 inch crepe pan or shallow nonstick skillet with oil. Heat over medium heat. Pour in 2 tablespoons of batter and tilt pan carefully so batter covers entire bottom of pan. Cook 2 minutes on each side or until golden brown. Repeat with remaining mixture, wiping pan or brushing with more oil, if needed.

Notes: Crepes are great filled with fresh fruit or sweetened and/or flavored whipped cream.

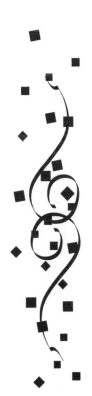

Quick Hints

Folding Crepes:
Blintz/Egg Roll

Place a portion of filling in the center of the crepe. Fold both side over about 1 inch. Roll from the bottom of the crepe, forming a cylindrical shape. The final product should resemble an egg roll.

Quesadilla

Spread one crepe with a portion of filling, then cover with second crepe. Cut into 6-8 wedges like a pizza. Great for appetizers!

Half Moon and Triangle

Spread one side of each crepe with a portion of filling. Fold the crepe in half (Half Moon).
For a triangle shape, fold in half again.

Cornucopia

Spread each crepe with a portion of filling and cut into quarters. Roll each quarter into a cone shape, thus looking like a cornucopia.

Roll/Foldover

Spoon a portion of filling in the center of each crepe, going edge to edge. Fold over one side to center, then the other making a neat packet. The filling should show at each end.

Cigarette/Roulade

Spread a portion of the filling over the surface, leaving a 1/2 inch border. Roll the crepe into a small cylinder or cigar. If desired, slice diagonally into thirds for appetizer-sized pieces.

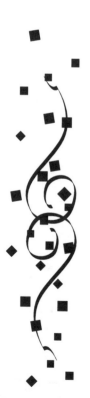

Envelope

Spoon a portion of filling in the center and fold both sides over to meet in the middle. Fold the top of the crepe down. Fold the bottom half up over both sides, making an envelope.

Purse

Place each crepe in a small ramekin and spoon in a portion of filling. Bring up the sides, forming pleats on top and tie with blanched green onion top or chive.

Cup

Place each crepe in a greased muffing cup or custard cup, carefully arranging the top in flutes. To fill after baking: place a small wad of foil in the crepe cup to keep the sides up, bake at 350°F for 10 minutes. If filled, bake at 350°F for 15 minutes. Great for desserts or appetizers.

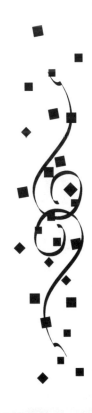

Crepes with Pear Butter

Serving Size: 8

8 Crepes
1 cup very ripe peeled pears, cored and cubed
1 cup butter, softened
1/4 cup maltitol, honey flavored

Spread about 1-1/2 tablespoons Honey-Pear Butter evenly over surface of hot crepes; fold crepes in quarters and serve immediately.

Place pear in a food processor or blender and blend until pureed. Add butter and maltitol and process until completely smooth. Spread about 1-1/2 tablespoons of mixture evenly over surface of hot crepes; fold crepes in quarters and serve immediately.

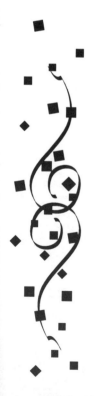

Lemon Pecan Scones

Serving Size: 16

3 cups all-purpose flour
1 tbsp baking powder
1/2 tsp salt
6 tbsps butter
1 1/4 cups milk
1/3 cup maltitol
2 tbsps lemon zest, grated
1 tsp lemon extract, optional
1/2 cup chopped pecans

Preheat oven to 450°F and lightly spray a baking sheet with nonstick cooking spray, set aside. Combine dry ingredients then cut in butter with a pastry blender until the flour has a coarse cornmeal texture. Combine the milk with the maltitol and remaining ingredients and add to the dry mixture, stirring with a fork. Turn the dough out onto a lightly floured table and knead 3 times. Cut the dough in half and pat out each half to a 1/2 inch thick circle. Cut each circle into 8 pieces, making 16 wedges total. Place them all on the baking sheet, a little apart from each other. Brush the tops of the scones with beaten egg, if desired. Bake 10-15 minutes, or until they are golden brown.

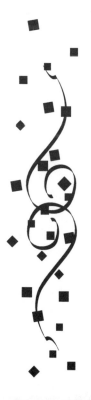

Linzer Dough

Serving Size: 8

1 1/2 cups all-purpose flour
1 cup hazelnuts, blanched and ground
3/4 cup maltitol
1 tsp cinnamon
1 tsp baking powder
12 tbsps unsalted butter, softened
1 egg
1 egg yolk
1/2 tsp lemon zest, grated
1/2 tbsp vanilla extract

Combine the flour, ground hazelnuts, cinnamon and baking powder, set aside. Mix the butter in a bowl until it is very soft, then gradually add the maltitol. Add the egg and egg yolk, one at a time, then the lemon zest and vanilla. By hand, mix in the flour mixture until the dough is smooth. Divide the dough in half and place each piece between two pieces of plastic wrap. Roll them out to about 1/4 inch thick, then refrigerate them until they are firm.

Notes: Almonds can be substituted for the hazelnuts.

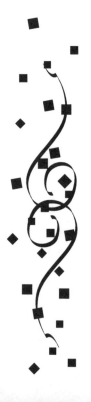

Linzertorte

Serving Size: 8

1 recipe Linzer dough *(recipe on page 190)*
20 ounces Raspberry all-fruit preserves, no sugar
    added

Preheat oven to 350°F. Roll out one piece of dough for bottom
of tart and press into the tart pan, leaving some dough
hanging over the edge. Stir the preserves until they are soft,
then place them in the tart pan over the dough. Roll out the
other piece of dough and place it on top of the tart, and seal
the edges as best as you can, removing the excess that hangs
over the edges. Cut a 1 inch hole in the middle of the tart so it
can vent and place it in the oven. Bake for 30 minutes, or, until
the crust is nicely browned. Let the tart cool in the pan before
removing it. Serve warm or at room temperature.

Notes: Apricot all-fruit preserves can be substituted for the
        raspberry preserves.

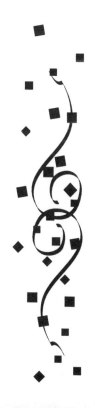

Mandeltorte

Serving Size: 8

1 recipe sweet tart dough *(recipe on page 265)*
1/2 cup butter
2 eggs
1/3 cup all-purpose flour
1/3 cup maltitol
1 tsp double-acting baking powder
1 cup shelled almonds ground
1 tsp almond extract
1/4 cup all-fruit raspberry preserves, no sugar added

Preheat oven to 350°F. Line tart pan with dough and press in. Soften butter and beat maltitol into it. Beat in eggs, one at a time, beating well between each. Stir in almonds and extract. Pour over pastry. Bake at 350°F for 30 minutes. Remove from oven and cool one hour. Spread jam over torte. Serve at room temperature with raspberry sauce.

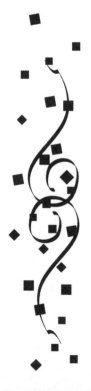

Pate Choux (Cream Puff Dough) ·

Serving Size: 12

8 tbsps unsalted butter
1 cup water
1/8 tsp salt
1 cup all-purpose flour
4 eggs at room temperature

Preheat oven to 400°F. Bring eater, salt and butter to a rolling boil over high heat. Add flour, all at once, to boiling mixture and turn down heat to medium. Stir in flour until it forms a ball, then stir it for 5 minutes more to cook out the starchy flavor. Remove from heat and place the dough in a bowl, beat with a mixer until the dough is almost room temperature. With mixer still on, add eggs one at a time, beating smooth after each addition. Drop dough by tablespoons onto a baking sheet that has been sprayed with nonstick cooking spray, each about 3 inches apart. Bake 20 minutes, then prick each shell with a toothpick to release air, and bake 10-15 minutes more, or until golden. Cool on a wire rack, then split puffs and fill with pastry cream or other filling.

Notes: To make eclairs, use a pastry bag with a plain tip and pipe out dough into 4 inch X 3/4 inch strips and bake the same as above.

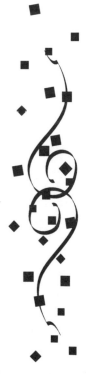

Sacher Torte

Serving Size: 10

1 recipe chocolate cake, cooked & cooled
   (recipe on page 66)
10 1/2 ounces apricot all-fruit preserves, no sugar
   added
1 recipe ganache, slightly warm *(recipe on page 270)*

Split the cake layers in half so that you have 4 equal layers. Mix the apricot preserves in a bowl a little to soften them, then spread it evenly between three layers. Place the last layer on top. Heat the ganache so that it is pourable, but not too thin. Set the cake on a rack and pour the ganache over the cake. Let the cake cool and the ganache harden somewhat, then serve.

Strawberries Romanoff

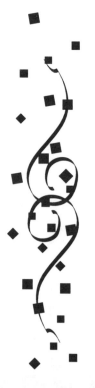

Serving Size: 4

1 1/2 quarts fresh strawberries, cleaned and halved
1/2 cup Cointreau
2 tbsps maltitol
1 cup heavy cream, whipped

Cover strawberries with maltitol and 2 tablespoons of Cointreau. Chill. Whip the cream and the remaining Cointreau until stiff. Pour the whipped bream over the strawberries and serve immediately.

Tea Scones

Serving Size: 12

3 cups all-purpose flour
1 tbsp baking powder
1/2 tsp salt
6 tbsps butter
1 1/4 cups milk
1/3 cup maltitol, honey flavored

Preheat oven to 450°F and lightly spray a baking sheet with nonstick cooking spray, set aside. Combine dry ingredients then cut in butter with a pastry blender until the flour has a coarse cornmeal texture. Combine the milk with the maltitol and add to the dry mixture, stirring with a fork. Turn the dough out onto a lightly floured table and knead 3 times. Cut the dough in half and pat out each half to a 1/2 inch thick circle. Cut each circle into 8 pieces, making 16 wedges total. Place them all on the baking sheet, a little apart from each other. Brush the tops of the scones with beaten egg, if desired. Bake 10-15 minutes, or until they are golden brown. These are great served with all-fruit preserves for breakfast.

Notes: 3/4 cup blueberries or raisins soaked in hot water can be added to the flour mixture before adding the liquid ingredients, both add lots of flavor.

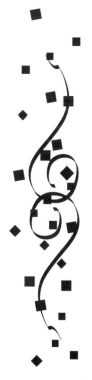

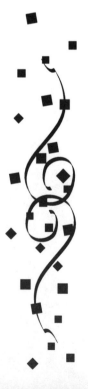

fruit
dishes

Apple and Almond Pocket

Serving Size: 6

1 1/3 cups all-purpose flour
1/2 tsp salt
1/2 cup butter
1 cup apples, sliced thin
3 tbsps brown sugar replacement
2 tbsps sliced almonds
1 recipe Apricot Glaze *(recipe on page 199)*

Preheat oven to 450°F. Sift the 1-1/3 cup flour with the salt
into a large mixing bowl. Cut in the butter with pastry blender
until mixture is the size of small peas. Sprinkle 4-5
tablespoons water, a little at a time, over the flour while
stirring with a fork, until mixture is just moist enough to hold
together. Form into a square and flatten to 1/2 inch. Roll out
on floured surface to 12 inch square. Place on ungreased
cookie sheet. Toss sliced apples with 1 tablespoon of flour.
Place slices down center third of dough. Sprinkle 2
tablespoons of brown sugar replacement over apples. Fold up
about 1/2 inch at each end. Fold sides over apples, leaving an
inch of apples showing down center. Sprinkle with 1
tablespoon brown sugar replacement and sliced almonds.
Bake for 15-20 minutes or until golden brown. Prepare apricot
glaze and brush over pastry immediately.

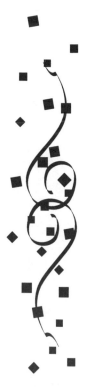

Apple Casserole

Serving Size: 8

3 cups Granny Smith apples, sliced
1/2 cup maltitol, honey flavored
1/4 tsp ground nutmeg
1/4 tsp ground cinnamon
1/8 tsp salt
Topping:
1 1/2 cups all-purpose flour
2 tsps baking powder
1/2 tsp salt
1/2 cup brown sugar replacement
1 large egg
1/2 cup milk
1/2 cup margarine, melted

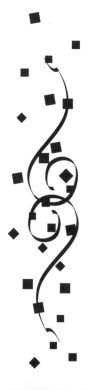

Preheat oven to 350°F. Spray a 1-1/2 quart casserole baking dish with nonstick cooking spray, set aside. Prepare apples. Place the apples in baking dish. Drizzle the maltitol over the apples and then sprinkle the spices over that. Bake until apples are soft. Pierce with a sharp knife to test when soft, increase oven temperature to 375°F, then pour the topping over apples and bake for 25 minutes longer or until top is brown and crusty.

TOPPING: Sift together the flour, baking powder, salt and sugar. Mix together the egg which has been well beaten, milk and melted margarine. Stir gently into the flour mixture. Pour over cooked apples and bake until crusty and browned.

Apple Cream Clouds

Serving Size: 6

6 large apples, quartered, unpeeled and cored
1/3 cup apple cider, no sugar added
1/2 cup maltitol, honey flavored
1/2 tsp lemon zest, grated
1/8 tsp nutmeg or cinnamon
1 cup whipping cream
1/4 cup maltitol

Place apple quarters in a heavy saucepan with cider and maltitol. Bring to a boil over medium heat, stirring to prevent scorching. Continue to cook and stir until apples become mushy. Puree through food mill and stir in spices and lemon zest. Cool.

While apple puree cools, beat cream until it forms stiff peaks. Gradually add maltitol and blend well. Fold 1/2 cup of apple puree into whipped cream, then fold whipped cream into remaining apple puree. Spoon into parfait glasses and chill thoroughly. Sprinkle top of each apple cream with nutmeg or cinnamon before serving.

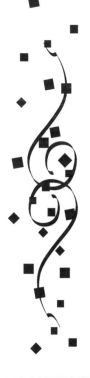

Apples with Calvados

Serving Size: 6

6 apples, medium size
3 tbsps lemon juice
3/4 cup Calvados or apple brandy
2 tbsps unsalted butter
apple cider, no sugar added

Preheat oven to 375°F and spray a 9X13 inch cooking dish lightly with nonstick cooking spray. Peel, core and slice the apples, then toss them in the lemon juice. Arrange the apple slices in a glass baking dish. Pour Calvados over the apples. Dot with the butter. Add enough apple cider to cover the apples. Bake for 20 minutes. Serve warm.

Baked Pear Gratin

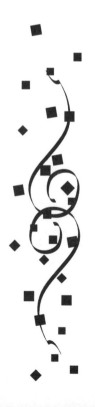

Serving Size: 6

4 medium pears
1 tbsp fresh lemon juice
2 tbsps dark rum
2 tbsps ground almonds
1/2 tsp cinnamon
1 tbsp date sugar

Preheat oven to 375°F and spray a 13X9X2 inch baking dish with nonstick cooking spray. Peel, core, and thinly slice pears and layer in bottom of baking dish. Sprinkle with lemon juice and rum. Combine almonds, cinnamon, and date sugar. Sprinkle over pears. Cover pan with aluminum foil and bake for 40 minutes. Remove aluminum foil and place pan under broiler. Broil to a light golden brown (3 to 5 minutes), and serve immediately.

Balsamic Marinated Strawberries

Serving Size: 4

1 pint strawberries, washed and quartered
1/4 cup balsamic vinegar
2 tbsps maltitol

Combine all ingredients in a plastic bag and marinate, refrigerated, overnight. Drain strawberries before serving and serve with a dollop of whipped cream.

Notes: Strawberries and vinegar sounded like an awful match when I first saw this recipe, but after I tried it, I was very impressed.

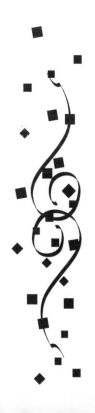

Blueberry Buckle

Serving Size: 6

1/4 cup margarine
1/2 cup maltitol, maple flavored
1 egg, beaten
1 cup all-purpose flour
1 1/2 tsps baking powder
1/8 tsp salt
1/3 cup milk
1 tsp vanilla extract
2 cups blueberries, unsweetened
Crumb topping:
1/2 cup brown sugar replacement
1/4 cup margarine
1/3 cup flour
1/2 tsp cinnamon

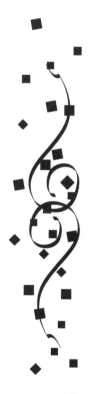

Preheat oven to 375°F. Cream margarine and maltitol together. Add well-beaten egg and mix together thoroughly. Sift flour, baking powder and salt together; add to creamed mixture alternately with milk and vanilla. Pour batter into an 8 x 8 inch pan that has been sprayed with nonstick cooking spray. Cover with blueberries. To make topping, cream margarine and brown sugar replacement, stir in flour and cinnamon until mixture is crumbly. Sprinkle crumb topping over blueberries.

Bake for 45 minutes or until done.

Broiled Grapefruit

Serving Size: 4

2 large ruby red grapefruits, segmented
1/4 tsp ginger
4 tbsps brown sugar replacement
2 tbsps warm water

Set oven to broil and cover a baking pan (or broiler pan) with foil. Combine ginger, brown sugar replacement and water and stir until smooth. Place grapefruit segments on baking tray and brush with mixture. Set under broiler 1-2 minutes or until hot and bubbly. Serve warm.

Figs with Creme Fraiche

Serving Size: 4

12 large figs, stems removed
1/4 cup orange liqueur
2 tbsps maltitol, honey flavored
1 recipe creme fraiche *(recipe on page 205)*

Slice figs into 6 wedges leaving to bottoms intact so that the figs look life a flower when the wedges are separated. Toss the figs with the orange liqueur. Combine the maltitol and creme fraiche. Place 3 figs on each plate and place a dollop of creme fraiche in the middle of each. Serve slightly chilled.

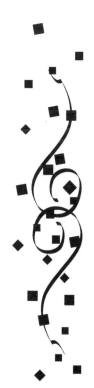

Grape Delight

Serving Size: 4

1/2 pound seedless grapes
1/2 cup vanilla yogurt, no sugar added
1/2 cup lowfat sour cream
1 tbsp maltitol
1/2 cup sliced almonds, toasted

Slice grapes in half and divide between 4 dessert glasses. Combine yogurt, sour cream and maltitol, stir until smooth and spoon over grapes. Top each glass with 2 tablespoons of almonds.

Honey-Baked Rum Bananas

Serving Size: 6

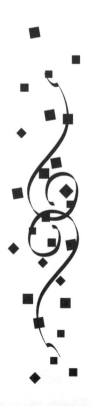

4 tbsps butter
6 bananas
2 tbsps fresh lemon juice
1/2 cup maltitol, honey flavored
1 1/2 tbsps dark rum
 dash ground cinnamon

Preheat oven to 350°F. Butter a baking dish with 1 tablespoon of the butter. Peel bananas and leave whole. Place in a single layer in the baking dish. Sprinkle with the lemon juice. Drizzle maltitol on top evenly and dot with remaining 3 tablespoons butter. Bake for about 20 minutes. Turn bananas once or twice as they are baking. Sprinkle with cinnamon. Just before serving, heat rum carefully and pour over bananas. Serve immediately.

Low Fat Raspberry and Pear Crisp

Serving Size: 10

1 1/2 cups sliced pears
2 cups fresh raspberries
1/4 cup dried currants, soaked in hot water
1/3 cup maltitol
2 tbsps cornstarch
1 tbsp lemon juice
1 tbsp grated lemon zest
1 cup rolled oats
3 tbsps melted unsalted butter
2 tbsps maltitol
1/2 tsp cinnamon
1/4 tsp cardamom

Preheat oven to 375°F and spray a 13X9X2 inch baking pan with nonstick cooking spray. Arrange pear slices in bottom of pan. Cover with raspberries, then currants. Mix together maltitol, cornstarch, lemon juice, and zest, and drizzle over pear mixture. In a large bowl combine oats, butter, maltitol, cinnamon, and cardamom. Crumble over pear mixture. Bake crisp until pears are tender and oats are lightly browned, about 30 to 40 minutes. Serve warm.

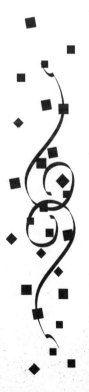

Marinated Pineapple

Serving Size: 4

1 medium pineapple
1/2 cup light rum
1/4 cup brown sugar replacement
 sweetened whipped cream

Prepare pineapple by first cutting off the top and bottom. Remove the hard outer skin and the eyes. Quarter the pineapple lengthwise, and remove the tough inner core. Dice the remaining pineapple into large chunks and combine with rum and brown sugar replacement in a plastic bag. Marinate for at least 2 hours, turning every hour or so. Drain pineapple before serving and serve with a dollop of whipped cream.

Minted Melons

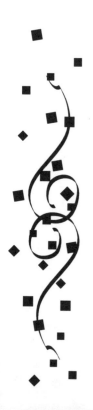

Serving Size: 6

1/2 small honeydew melon (2-1/2 to 3 pounds)
1 medium cantaloupe (1-3/4 to 2 pounds)
2 pounds watermelon wedge
1/4 cup maltitol, honey flavored
2 tbsps water
2 tbsps chopped fresh mint

Remove seeds from melons; cut into 1 inch balls. Place melon balls in a glass bowl. Combine maltitol, water and mint and mix well. Toss melon with mixture. Cover and refrigerate for 2 to 3 hours to blend flavors.

Sauteed Bananas

Serving Size: 4

2 tbsps butter
3 tbsps brown sugar replacement
1/4 cup orange juice
1 tbsp dark rum
1/8 tsp ground cinnamon
2 bananas
 sugar free ice cream

Melt butter in a medium skillet. Stir in brown sugar replacement, orange juice, rum, and cinnamon. Bring to a boil; cook and stir over medium-high heat for several minutes, or until mixture is reduced by about one quarter. Sauce will be slightly syrupy.

Peel bananas, split in half lengthwise, then slice bananas crosswise into 1 inch chunks. Add bananas to sauce in pan. Cook bananas just enough to heat through, basting with sauce. Spoon bananas and sauce over ice cream. Serve immediately.

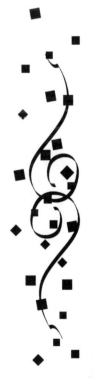

Wine Poached Pears

Serving Size: 6

6 large pears
2 tbsps fresh lemon juice
2 cups red wine
2 tsps cinnamon
1/2 tsp nutmeg
1 cup fresh orange juice

Peel whole pears then core them from the bottom (a melon baller makes this easier) leaving the pears whole. Add remaining ingredients to a sauce pot and bring to a boil - this will cook the alcohol out of the wine, Add pears and reduce to a simmer. Cook pears for about 30 minutes or until they are fork tender. Serve warm or chilled.

Notes: It is important for the pears to be completely submerged in the poaching liquid to ensure even cooking and coloring. If liquid doesn't cover the pears completely, double the poaching liquid recipe.

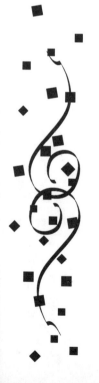

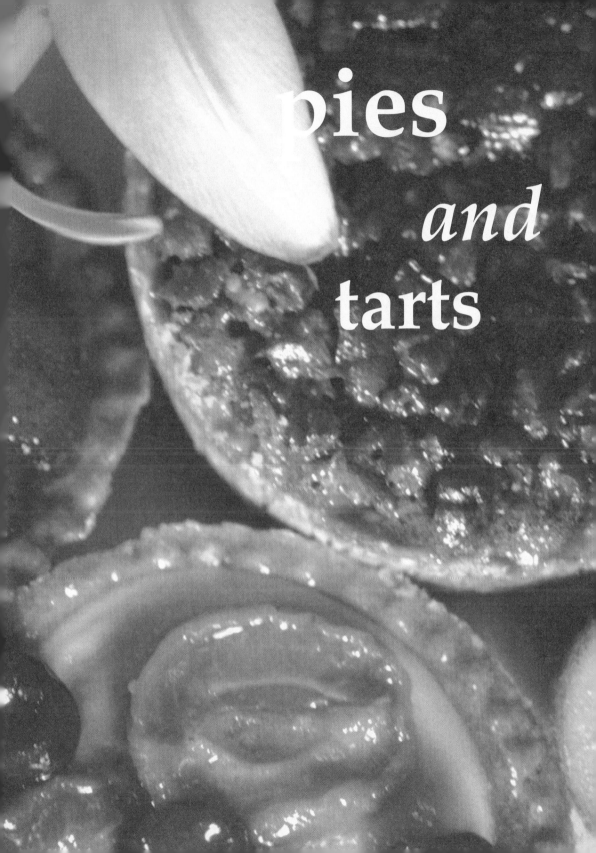

pies *and* tarts

Apple Pie

Serving Size: 8

2 pieces pie dough for double crust
6 cups peeled apples, cored and diced
1/4 cup maltitol
1 tbsp cornstarch
1 tsp cinnamon
1/4 tsp allspice

Preheat oven to 375°F. Divide dough for pie into two equal
balls, then roll them both out. Line a 9 inch pie pan with one
piece of crust, and reserve the other for the top. Mix together
all other ingredients and fill pie with it, pressing down to pack
apples in. Carefully lay top crust over pie and seal edges by
pressing down on them with fingers or a fork. Cut off or flute
any remaining pie dough that happens to hang over the edge.
Cut 4 slits on top of the crust. Bake pie for 50-60 minutes or
until crust is golden and inside is bubbly. Serve warm or
chilled.

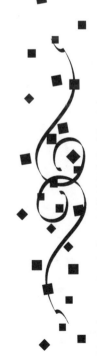

Blueberry Pie

Serving Size: 8

1 recipe pie dough for a double crusted pie
    (recipe on page 263)
4 cups blueberries
4 tsps lemon juice
3/4 cup maltitol
2 tbsps cornstarch
1 tsp lemon peel, grated
1/2 tsp ground cinnamon
1/8 tsp salt
2 tbsps butter

Preheat oven to 450°F and line a 9 inch pie tin with pie dough, have the other half rolled out, set aside. Sort, rinse and drain blueberries. Sprinkle lemon juice over berries. Combine maltitol, flour, lemon peel, and cinnamon. Toss this mixture gently with the blueberries to coat well. Put berry mixture into pie shell; dot with butter. Place second crust on top of pie, seal edges and cut a few slashes in top to allow steam to escape. Bake in preheated for 10 minutes. Lower heat to 350°F and continue baking 30-35 minutes more. Cool pie before slicing.

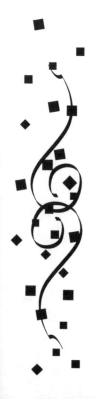

Buttermilk-Lemon Pie

Serving Size: 6

1 1/2 cups maltitol
3 tbsps all-purpose flour
1/4 tsp nutmeg
1/2 cup butter, melted
1 cup buttermilk
3 large eggs
1 lemon
1 9 inch pie crust, unbaked

Blend flour and nutmeg. Add maltitol and melted butter and beat until creamy. Add eggs one at a time, beating well after each. Mix in the buttermilk and lemon. Pour into unbaked 9-inch pie crust. Bake at 400°F for 10 minutes. Lower temperature to 325°F and continue baking for 30 minutes longer.

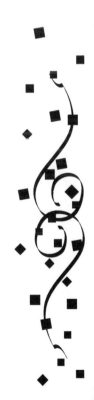

Butterscotch Cream Pie

Serving Size: 8

1 recipe pie crust (9 inch), baked and cooled
     (recipe on page 264)
2 1/2 cups milk
2/3 cup brown sugar replacement
1/8 tsp salt
1/3 cup cornstarch
3 eggs, well beaten
4 tbsps unsalted butter, softened
2 tsps vanilla extract

Bake pie crust and set aside to cool. Combine milk, brown
sugar replacement, salt and cornstarch and bring to boil in a
heavy saucepan over medium heat. Stir frequently to avoid
scorching the bottom. When mixture boils, add about 1 cup of
the hot liquid to the egg yolks and mix until combined. Add
the yolk mixture to the pan and reduce heat to low (do not
boil again). Cook for 5 minutes more or until the mixture is
very thick. Remove from the heat and stir in butter and
vanilla. Pour into prepared pie crust and refrigerate. Allow
pie to cool completely before serving.

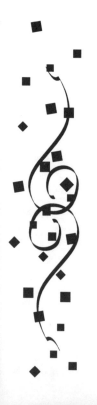

Butterscotch Pie

Serving Size: 8

3 tbsps butter
2 cups brown sugar replacement
2 cups milk
3 eggs
1/4 cup all-purpose flour
1/2 tsp salt
1 1/4 tsps vanilla extract
1 9 inch pie crust, baked
3 tbsps maltitol

Place butter in a heavy saucepan over medium heat. Heat
until melted. Add brown sugar replacement and 1/2 cup
milk; mix well. Bring to a boil and cook for 5 minutes, stirring
constantly. Beat the egg yolks; stir in remaining milk.
Combine flour and salt; stir egg mixture into this. Add small
amount of the hot brown sugar mix gradually. Stir and return
this to the mixture in skillet. Cook over low heat, stirring
constantly, until thickened. Cool slightly and blend in 1
teaspoon vanilla. Pour into pre-baked pie crust. Preheat oven
to 325°F. Beat egg whites until stiff peaks form; slowly add
maltitol. Fold in the remaining 1/4 teaspoon vanilla. Pile this
on top of pie, sealing to edges. Bake for about 10-15 minutes
or until lightly browned. Serve warm or cold.

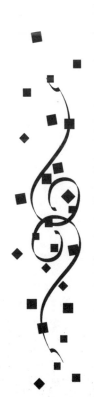

Cherry Pie

Serving Size: 8

1 recipe pie crust for double crusted pies
  (recipe on page 263)
1 cup maltitol
1/3 cup all-purpose flour
5 cups cherries in water or fresh, pitted
1/2 tsp almond extract

Preheat oven to 375°F and prepare pie dough for pie. Line pie tin with 1/2 of crust and roll out the other half to have ready. Combine maltitol, flour and cherries and toss until everything is evenly dispersed. Pour cherry mixture into prepared pie tin. Place other crust on top, seal the edges and trim off excess crust. Cut a hole in the middle of the pie so the steam can vent. Place in the oven and bake 50 - 60 minutes, or until filling is bubbly. If pie gets too dark while cooking, place a piece of foil very loosely on top of the pie. Serve warm or chilled.

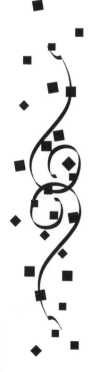

Chocolate Cream Pie

Serving Size: 8

1/4 cup cornstarch or arrowroot
1 dash salt
2 ounces unsweetened chocolate squares, chopped fine
3 cups milk
3 egg yolks, slightly beaten
2 tbsps butter
1 tsp vanilla extract
5 1/2 tsps Equal® sweetener
1 pie crust (9 inch) baked

Combine cornstarch (or arrowroot), salt, chocolate, and milk in a heavy bottomed saucepan and stir over medium heat until boiling gently. Turn heat to low and stir 1/2 cup of the hot milk mixture into the egg yolks and then return all to pan. Cook for about 3 more minutes (do not boil again) stirring constantly, until very thick and smooth. Remove from the heat and stir in vanilla and butter. Let cool 15 minutes, then stir in the Equal until it is all dissolved. Pour the filling into the pre-baked crust and refrigerate. Allow pie to cool completely before serving.

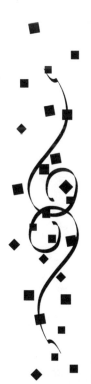

Chocolate Meringue Pie

Serving Size: 8

1 9 inch pie crust, baked
1 1/4 cups maltitol
3 tbsps unsweetened cocoa powder, sifted
1 1/2 cups milk
4 egg yolks
4 tbsps all-purpose flour
1 tsp vanilla extract
4 tbsps butter
 Meringue
4 egg whites
1/2 cup maltitol
1 pinch cream of tartar
1/2 tsp vanilla

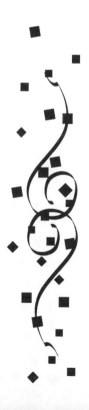

Beat egg yolks. Mix maltitol, flour, cocoa and milk together. Blend and add to egg yolks. Chip up the butter into small pieces and add to the egg mixture; add vanilla and blend. Bring to boil over medium heat, stirring constantly. Lower heat and cook 5 minutes. Pour into baked pie crust. In large mixing bowl, combine egg whites and pinch of cream of tartar. Beat until stiff but not dry. Add 1/2 teaspoon vanilla extract. Mix 1/2 cup maltitol gradually into egg whites. Beat well for at least five minutes, as mixing too little will cause the meringue to separate. Spread on top of pie, sealing to edges. Bake for few minutes at 350°F until meringue is light golden brown. Cool a few minutes before slicing.

Notes: To cut meringues perfectly every time, run the knife under warm water and then slice through the pie. Repeat this process for each slice you cut.

Chocolate Pecan Pie

Serving Size: 8

3 eggs beaten
1 1/4 cups maltitol
1/2 cup brown sugar replacement
3 ounces unsweetened chocolate squares, melted
2 tbsps margarine, melted
1 tsp vanilla extract
1 1/2 cups pecans, chopped
1 9 inch pie crust, unbaked

Preheat oven to 350°F. In a large bowl, mix eggs, maltitol, brown sugar replacement, melted chocolate, butter and vanilla until well blended. Blend in pecans. Pour into 9-inch unbaked pie shell. Bake for 50 to 60 minutes or until knife inserted halfway between center and edge comes out clean. Cool on wire rack.

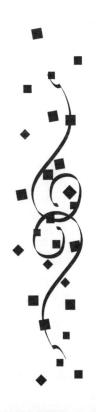

Coconut Cream Pie

Serving Size: 8

1/4 cup cornstarch or arrowroot
1 dash salt
3 cups milk
3 egg yolks, slightly beaten
3/4 cup coconut flakes, unsweetened
2 tbsps butter
1 tsp vanilla extract
5 1/4 tsps Equal® sweetener
1 pie crust (9 inch), baked

Toast 1/4 cup of the coconut for about 8 minutes in a 350°F oven until it is a golden color, set aside. Combine cornstarch (or arrowroot), salt and milk in a heavy bottomed saucepan and stir over medium heat until boiling gently. Turn heat to low and stir 1/2 cup of the hot milk mixture into the egg yolks and then return all to pan. Cook for about 3 more minutes (do not boil again) stirring constantly, until very thick and smooth. Remove from the heat and stir in coconut, vanilla and butter. Let cool 15 minutes, then stir in the Equal until it is all dissolved. Pour the filling into the pre-baked crust, sprinkle with toasted coconut and refrigerate. Allow pie to cool completely before serving.

Notes: Unsweetened coconut can be found in natural food stores.

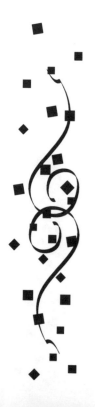

Cottage Cheese Pie

Serving Size: 8

2 cups lowfat cottage cheese
3 large eggs
1/2 cup maltitol
1/2 cup cream
1/2 tsp ground cinnamon
1 tbsp lemon zest, grated
1 tbsp fresh lemon juice
1 9 inch pie crust

Preheat oven to 425°F and line pie pan with pie dough, set aside. Mix cottage cheese, eggs, maltitol and milk. Use wire whisk to blend thoroughly. Add remaining ingredients and blend. Pour into unbaked crust. Bake for 10 minutes. Lower heat to 350°F and continue baking for 20-25 minutes longer. Allow pie to cool before slicing.

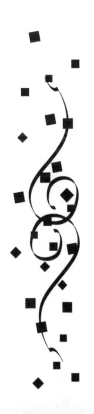

Cream Cheese-Lemon Pie

Serving Size: 8

1 9 inch pie crust baked for 10 minutes
1/2 cup maltitol
1 dash salt
12 ounces cream cheese
1/2 cup lemon juice
2 large eggs
1 cup sour cream
1 tbsp lemon zest, not dried

In a mixing bowl, combine cream cheese and lemon juice; blend well. Add eggs and maltitol; beat very well with a wire whisk until smooth. Pour into crust. Bake in preheated 350°F oven for 20 minutes or until firm. Remove from oven and let cool only 5 minutes. Mix sour cream, lemon zest and 3-4 tablespoons sugar. Spread this mixture over pie filling; bake 10 minutes more. Cool for a few minutes then refrigerate and chill 4-6 hours before serving.

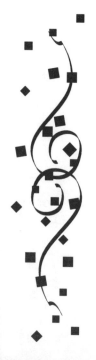

Fresh Strawberry Pie

Serving Size: 8

1 9 inch pie crust, baked
3 pints strawberries
1 cup maltitol
3 tbsps cornstarch
1 tbsp butter

Wash and drain strawberries very well. Place 2/3 of the strawberries in a baked pie shell. Arrange decoratively. Crush the remaining 1 pint of strawberries; add maltitol, cornstarch, butter, and 1/2 cup water in a saucepan. Cook the mixture until thick, stirring often. Pour over whole berries in pie shell. Let cool a few minutes, then refrigerate. Serve with whipped cream, if desired.

Fresh Strawberry-Rhubarb Pie

Serving Size: 8

2 cups rhubarb, diced
1 pint strawberries, washed and dried
3/4 cup maltitol
2 tbsps tapioca, quick-cooking
3 tbsps butter
1 recipe pie crust for double crusted pie
   (recipe on page 263)

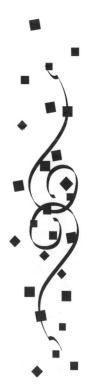

Preheat oven to 375°F. Wash rhubarb, cut away any tough parts and chop into small pieces. Slice the strawberries and add to rhubarb. Mix the maltitol and tapioca and add to fruit. Blend well and allow to stand for 15 minutes to allow syrup to penetrate strawberries. Pour mixture into unbaked 9-inch pie crust, dot with butter and cover with second crust. Cut slits in top crust. Bake for 50-55 minutes. Cover pie with aluminum foil tented over it if it browns too quickly.

Kahlua Pecan Pie

Serving Size: 8

3/4 cup maltitol
3 eggs
1 tsp vanilla extract
3/4 cup pecan halves
1 9 inch pie crust
1/2 cup heavy whipping cream
2 tbsps Kahlua

Beat the eggs slightly and add the maltitol, vanilla and halves of pecans; blend well. Pour into unbaked pie shell. Bake in a preheated 325°F oven for 45 minutes. Cool on wire rack. To make the topping, mix the whipping cream and the liqueur. Beat until peaks form. Serve immediately, placing a dollop of cream on each slice of pie.

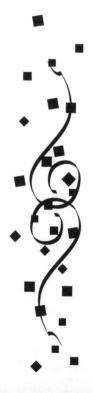

Lemon Cream Pie

Serving Size: 8

1 pie crust (9 inch), baked
4 egg yolks
1 1/2 tbsps lemon zest, grated
3 tbsps fresh lemon juice
1 cup heavy cream
3 1/2 tsps Equal® sweetener

Combine egg yolks, lemon zest, and lemon juice and beat until light and lemon colored. Place this mixture in a heat proof glass bowl then set the bowl on top of a saucepan of simmering water (this will gently cook the mixture). While the bowl is over the water, stir constantly until mixture is very thick and clings to a wooden spoon. Remove from the heat and let cool to room temperature. Pour cream and Equal into a chilled bowl and beat until medium peaks form. Fold cream into lemon mixture, pour into crust and refrigerate 24 hours before serving. This pie is great when topped with sweetened whipped cream, or for an especially elegant dessert, leave off the cream and top with fresh raspberries.

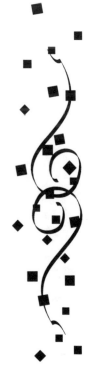

Meringue For Pie

Serving Size: 8

4 egg whites at room temperature
1 tsp vanilla extract
1/2 tsp cream of tartar
1/2 cup maltitol

This recipe is good for any single crusted pie that you would like to make into a meringue pie. The pie should already have a baked crust and cooked filling.

Preheat oven to 350°F. Whip the egg whites and cream of tartar until they look foamy. Gradually add maltitol and whip to soft peaks. Add vanilla and whip to stiff peaks. Spread meringue over pie making sure it touches the entire edge of the pie (this keeps it from shrinking). Bake for about 15 minutes or until the meringue is the color you like.

Notes: Meringues are especially good on chocolate and lemon cream pies.

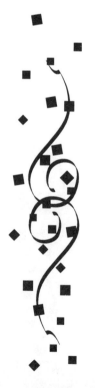

Peach Crumb-Top Pie

Serving Size: 8

3 tbsps all-purpose flour
1/3 cup maltitol
1/4 tsp ground cinnamon
3 cups peach slices
Topping:
2 tbsps butter
1/3 cup rolled oats
1/2 cup brown sugar replacement
1/3 cup all-purpose flour
1/4 tsp ground cinnamon
1 9 inch pie crust

Preheat oven to 375°F. In a mixing bowl, combine flour, maltitol, cinnamon, stir in peaches and toss to coat well. Place mixture into unbaked pie shell. In a small bowl, combine all topping ingredients and cut in butter with a pastry blender or two knives until mixture is crumbly. Sprinkle evenly over top of fruit in pie shell. Place a baking sheet on oven rack; set pie atop the sheet. Bake for about 40 minutes or until golden brown.

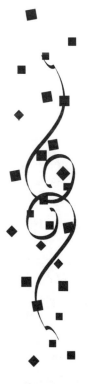

Peanut Butter Pie

Serving Size: 8

1 cup chunky peanut butter, no sugar added
1 tsp vanilla extract
2 tbsps butter, melted
3 large eggs, slightly beaten
1 cup maltitol
1/2 cup brown sugar replacement
1 9 inch pie crust
 whipped cream

Preheat oven to 450°F and line a pie tin with pie crust, set aside. Combine peanut butter, vanilla and melted butter in bowl. Blend well. In large bowl place the eggs, maltitol and brown sugar replacement. Beat until thoroughly combined. Stir the 2 mixtures together until completely blended. Pour into the pie shell and bake for 10 minutes; lower temperature to 325°F and bake for 35-40 minutes longer, or until firm to the touch. Cool on wire rack. Serve warm or chilled with sweetened whipped cream, if desired.

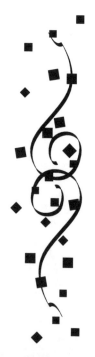

Pineapple Pie

Serving Size: 8

8 1/2 ounces crushed pineapple, well drained
1/3 cup margarine
1/2 cup brown sugar replacement
3/4 cup maltitol
3 large eggs
1 tsp vanilla extract
1 9 inch pie crust

Preheat oven to 350°F and line a pie tin with pie dough, set
aside. Cream butter and brown sugar replacement together
until light and fluffy. While mixing, gradually add maltitol.
Add eggs one at a time, beating well after each addition. Add
vanilla extract and drained pineapple; blend. Pour into
unbaked pie shell and bake for about 45 minutes. Let cool for
a few minutes before cutting, or serve cold.

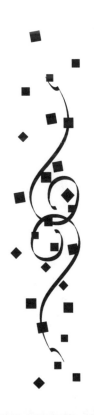

Spicy Carrot Pie

Serving Size: 8

1 cup shredded carrots
1/2 cup dates, chopped fine
1/2 cup brown sugar replacement
1 tbsp flour
1/2 tsp ground cinnamon
1/4 tsp ground ginger
1/4 tsp ground nutmeg
1/8 tsp ground cloves
1 egg
3/4 cup evaporated milk
1 9 inch pie crust
Topping:
1/3 cup brown sugar replacement
1/4 cup dried coconut, unsweetened
1/4 cup pecans, chopped
2 tbsps butter
1 1/2 tbsps evaporated milk

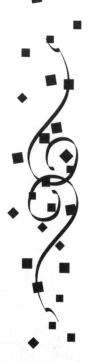

Combine the grated carrots, dates, brown sugar replacement, flour, and all the spices. Mix to blend. Add the beaten egg and evaporated milk, blend well. Pour into unbaked pie shell. Preheat oven to 425°F and bake the pie for 10 minutes. Lower heat to 350 and bake 25 minutes longer, or until knife inserted 1/3 in from edge comes out clean. Make topping by blending all the topping ingredients together. Remove from oven and sprinkle topping over pie. Place under the broiler for 2-3 minutes or until bubbling and golden brown. Serve topped with sweetened whipped cream if desired.

Notes: Be sure to use evaporated milk and not condensed milk, the latter is loaded with sugar!

Vanilla Cream Pie

Serving Size: 8

1/4 cup cornstarch or arrowroot
1 dash salt
3 cups milk
3 egg yolks, slightly beaten
2 tbsps butter
1 1/2 tsps vanilla extract
5 1/4 tsps Equal® sweetener
1 pie crust (9 inch) baked

Combine cornstarch (or arrowroot), salt and milk in a heavy
bottomed saucepan and stir over medium heat until boiling
gently. Turn heat to low and stir 1/2 cup of the hot milk
mixture into the egg yolks and then return all to pan. Cook
for about 3 more minutes (do not boil again) stirring
constantly, until very thick and smooth. Remove from the heat
and stir in vanilla and butter. Let cool 15 minutes, then stir in
the Equal until it is all dissolved. Pour the filling into the pre-
baked crust, and refrigerate. Allow pie to cool completely
before serving.

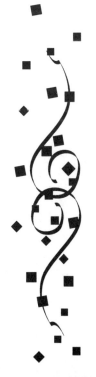

Black Bottom Raspberry Tart

Serving Size: 8

1 recipe chocolate tart dough *(recipe on page 261)*
1 ounce unsweetened chocolate, chopped
2 tbsps maltitol
1 recipe pastry cream
1 pint fresh raspberries

Preheat oven to 325°F. Roll out tart dough and press it into tart pan. Prick ALL over with a fork and bake for 20 minutes. Set aside to let cool. Combine chocolate and maltitol in a small bowl. Microwave 30 seconds at a time until chocolate is melted, stirring each time. When chocolate is melted, mix it well with the syrup and pour it into the tart crust. Spread the chocolate so that it covers the entire bottom. Once chocolate has hardened, spoon pastry cream into the shell and make it so that it is flush with the top of the crust. Carefully place raspberries on top of pastry cream, covering every space. Raspberry topped tarts do not require an apricot glaze. Refrigerate before serving.

Notes: When using raspberries, I prefer to brush them gently instead of washing them because once they are exposed to moisture, they tend to mold quickly.

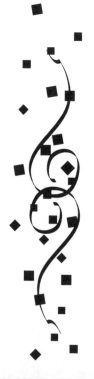

Fresh Fruit Tart

Serving Size: 8

1 recipe sweet tart dough, baked *(recipe on page 265)*
1 recipe pastry cream recipe *(recipe on page 259)*
6 large strawberries, washed and dried
1/2 cup raspberries
2 kiwi fruit, peeled
1/2 cup orange sections
1 recipe apricot glaze

After the tart shell has baked and cooled off, spoon the pastry cream into the shell and smooth the top so it is flat - the cream should be even with the top of the crust. Cut the strawberries and kiwi into thin slices, discard the end pieces. You can place the fruit on the tart any way you like, but here is a suggestion that works well: place the strawberry slices on the outermost edge with the tip of the strawberries facing inward, all around the tart. Next, place the kiwi slices just inside the strawberries, with each piece of fruit overlapping the other just a little. In the center, arrange the orange segments so that they form a fan, each piece facing the same direction. Place raspberries anywhere that you can see pastry cream - there will probably be spaces between the strawberries and kiwi. Once you have finished placing the fruit, prepare the apricot glaze and brush the top of the tart with it. Refrigerate the tart until serving time.

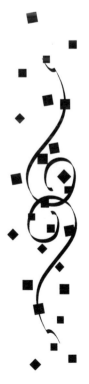

Lemon Custard Tart

Serving Size: 8

1 recipe sweet tart dough *(recipe on page 265)*
grated rind of 1 small lemon
juice of 2 medium lemons
1/2 cup maltitol, honey flavored
2 eggs
1 recipe apricot glaze *(recipe on page 266)*

Preheat oven to 325°F. Roll out tart dough and press into tart pan. Prick ALL over with a fork and bake for 10 minutes. Set aside to cool, increase temperature to 350°F. In a blender or food processor, combine lemon rind, juice, maltitol, and eggs, and puree until smooth. Pour lemon filling into prepared tart and bake for about 30-40 minutes, or until crust is golden and tart is lightly browned. If you would like an unusual looking tart, turn the broiler on and place tart under it, rotating as necessary until the top is covered with dark brown spots. Glaze with apricot glaze.

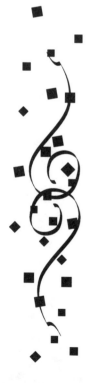

Peach Pistachio Tart

Serving Size: 8

1 recipe Nutty Tart Crust made with pistachios
    (recipe on page 262)
2 pounds canned peaches in fruit juice
3/4 cup pistachio nuts, skinned
1 tsp almond extract
1/2 cup maltitol
2 eggs
4 tbsps unsalted butter
1/4 cup all-purpose flour

Roll out dough for tart pan and press it into the pan. Prick
dough with a fork ALL over, then bake it 10 minutes in an
oven preheated to 325°F, set aside. Drain peaches and cut
them so that they fan out some, set aside. Place pistachios in a
food processor and pulse until they are finely ground. Place
the pistachio mixture in a bowl and add almond extract,
maltitol and one of the eggs while mixing at medium speed.
Add the other egg, mix in completely, them add the butter.
After the butter is incorporated, scrape down the sides and
add the flour. Mix in the flour just until no flour particles
show. Spread this filling in the prebaked tart shell so that it is
flat on top. Arrange peaches over the top of the filling. Place
tart in oven and bake for about 45 minutes more - the tart is
done when a toothpick inserted in the filling part comes out
clean. Glaze tart with apricot glaze before serving.

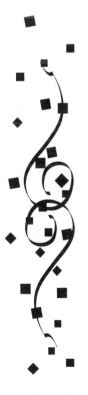

Pear Pecan Tart

Serving Size: 8

1 recipe Nutty Tart Crust made with pecans
        (*recipe on page 262*)
2 pounds pears, canned in juice
1 cup pecans
1/2 tsp cinnamon
1/2 cup brown sugar replacement
2 tsps vanilla extract
2 eggs
4 tbsps unsalted butter, softened.
1/4 cup all-purpose flour
1 recipe Apricot Glaze (*recipe on page 266*)

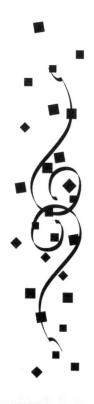

Roll out dough for tart pan and press it into the pan. Prick dough with a fork ALL over, then bake it 10 minutes in an oven preheated to 325°F, set aside. Drain pears and cut them so that they fan out some, set aside. Combine pecans, cinnamon and brown sugar replacement in a food processor and pulse until mixture is finely ground. Place the pecan mixture in a bowl and add vanilla and one of the eggs while mixing at medium speed. Add the other egg, mix in completely, them add the butter. After the butter is incorporated, scrape down the sides and add the flour. Mix in the flour just until no flour particles show. Spread this filling in the prebaked tart shell so that it is flat on top. Arrange pears over the top of the filling. Place tart in oven and bake for about 45 minutes more - the tart is done when a toothpick inserted in the filling part comes out clean. Glaze tart with apricot glaze before serving.

Plum Tart

Serving Size: 8

1 recipe Nutty Tart Crust made with almonds
    (recipe on page 262)
2 eggs
1/2 cup chopped almonds
8 medium plums, halved and pitted
1/4 cup sour cream
1 tbsp maltitol

Preheat oven to 350°F. Roll out tart dough and press into tart pan and sprinkle with chopped almonds. Place halved plums on top. Beat together eggs, sour cream and maltitol. Pour filling over plums. Bake for 1-1/4 hours, then brown at 375°F for 10 minutes.

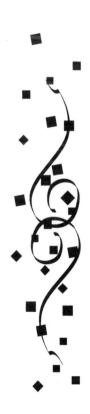

Strawberry Tart

Serving Size: 8

1 recipe sweet tart dough, baked *(recipe on page 265)*
1 recipe pastry cream
1 pint fresh strawberries, washed and dried
1 recipe Apricot Glaze *(recipe on page 266)*

After the tart shell has been baked and cooled, spoon the
pastry cream into the shell and smooth it out so that the cream
is even with the top of the crust. Slice the strawberries into
1/8 inch slices, discard the end pieces. Place the strawberries
on the tart starting from the outer edge and working your
way in. Place the berries pointed tip inwards, and layer them
slightly so that no pastry cream can be seen in between them.
After the tart is covered with the berries, prepare the glaze
and brush over the top of the tart lightly. Refrigerate until
served.

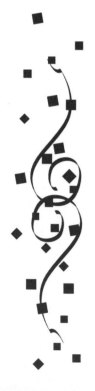

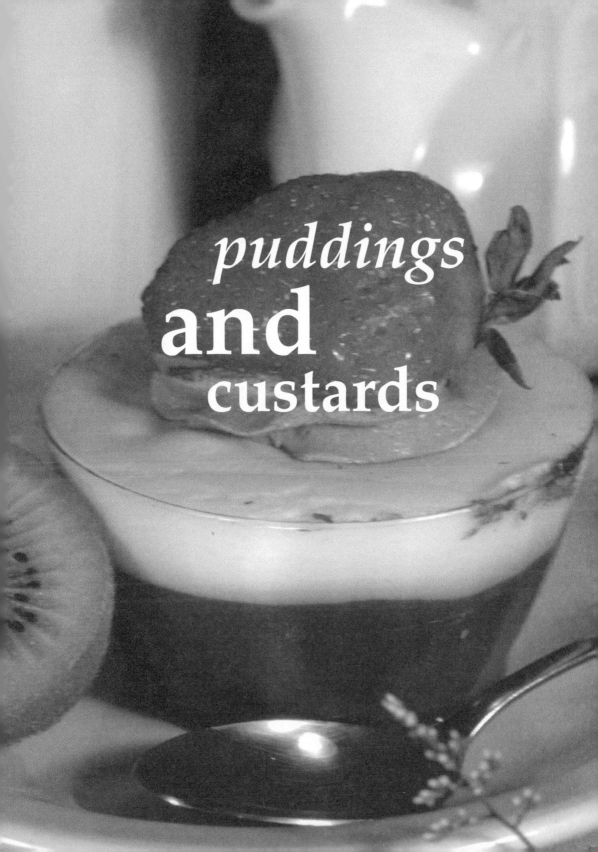

puddings and custards

Apple and Pecan Bread Pudding

Serving Size: 12

12 slices (about 3/4 in. thick) French bread
1/2 cup butter, melted
4 cups half-and-half
3/4 cup maltitol
1/2 cup brown sugar replacement
5 eggs
1 tsp vanilla extract
1 pinch salt
4 large golden delicious apples, peeled & sliced
    thin
1 cup toasted pecan halves

Preheat oven to 425°F and brush bread with some of the melted butter. Put bread slices on a baking sheet and bake until golden brown (about 10 minutes). In a medium saucepan over medium-low heat, bring half-and-half to a simmer (bubbles will appear at edge of pan). In a 3-quart bowl, beat maltitol and brown sugar replacement with eggs; whisk hot half-and-half into egg-sugar mixture. Stir in vanilla and salt; set aside. Pour remaining butter into a 9- by 12 inch baking dish. Place 6 bread slices in dish; strain half of egg-custard mixture through a wire mesh strainer over bread. Distribute sliced apples over bread-custard mixture; top with pecans. Arrange remaining bread over fruit and strain remaining egg-custard mixture over bread. Let stand 1 hour, covered with plastic wrap. Preheat oven to 325°F. Bake, uncovered, until golden brown and slightly crusty (about 1-3/4 hours). Serve warm.

Notes: This bread pudding goes great with creme anglaise, cinnamon sauce or sweetened whipped cream.

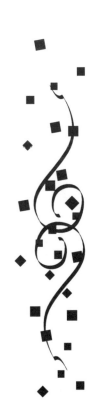

Best Ever Rice Pudding

Serving Size: 6

3 cups skim milk
1/3 cup long-grain rice
1/3 cup currants
1/4 cup brown sugar replacement
1 tsp vanilla extract
 dash cinnamon

In a heavy bottomed saucepan, bring milk to a boil, then stir in rice and currants. Turn heat to low and cover. Cook until rice absorbs most of the milk and is tender, about 30 minutes. Stir in brown sugar replacement and vanilla and spoon into serving dishes. Give the top of each a dash of cinnamon. Best when served warm.

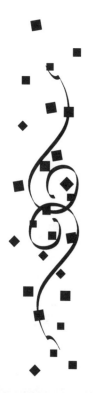

Chevre Custard

Serving Size: 4

1 large egg
1/3 cup maltitol
1 tsp cornstarch
1 1/2 tsps fresh lemon juice
1 tsp vanilla extract
1 pound creamy chevre cheese
1/4 cup milk

Preheat oven to 375°F and lightly spray four custard cups with nonstick cooking spray, set aside. Combine first five ingredients in a large bowl and mix until well combined without whipping too much air into the mixture. Combine chevre and milk and mix until smooth then add to the egg mixture, stirring until smooth. Strain mixture. Pour into prepared custard cups and place the cups in a larger pan that will fit all the cups. Pour one inch of hot water in the larger pan. Bake for 10 minutes then reduce the oven temperature to 325°F. Bake about 35 more minutes or until the custard is almost set. Let custards cool to room temperature then cover and refrigerate overnight. Serve with apricot sauce or any other fruit sauce.

Notes: Chevre cheese is a cheese made from goat milk - it can usually be found in most delis.

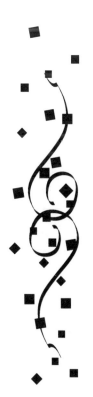

Chocolate Bread Pudding

Serving Size: 4

1 1/2 cups skim milk
1 cup maltitol
1 cup soft bread crumbs
1 1/2 ounces unsweetened chocolate squares
2 tbsps margarine
2 large eggs
1/4 tsp salt
1/2 tsp vanilla extract
1/2 cup skim milk
 sweetened whipped cream

Place in top of double boiler the 1-1/2 cups milk, maltitol, stale bread crumbs and chocolate. Cook over hot water until smooth. Stir in 2 tablespoons margarine. Beat eggs until light; add salt, vanilla and 1/2 cup milk. Whisk into the chocolate mixture. Cook until thick. Pour into a casserole dish that has been sprayed with nonstick cooking spray and bake for 20 minutes at 350°F. Serve warm or chill and serve with whipped cream.

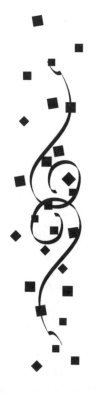

Chocolate Cinnamon Custard

Serving Size: 4

1 1/2 cups half and half
1 ounce unsweetened chocolate squares, chopped
1/2 cup maltitol
1 tsp vanilla
1/2 tsp cinnamon
3 eggs

Preheat oven to 325°F and place 4 custard cups in a larger baking dish, set aside. In a heavy saucepan, combine half and half, chocolate and maltitol over medium heat. Stir constantly until half and half comes to a simmer and chocolate is melted. Add the vanilla and cinnamon to the mixture. In a separate bowl, beat the eggs without incorporating too much air into them. Add the chocolate mixture to this and stir well. Strain custard and pour evenly into custard cups. Pour warm water 1/2 way up the sides of the cups and place in the oven. Bake for 30-40 minutes or until a knife inserted near the middle comes out clean. Remove from water bath and chill until service.

Notes: Cinnamon can be omitted, if desired.

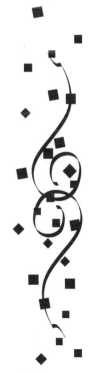

Coconut Mousse

Serving Size: 8

8 ounces lowfat cream cheese, softened
1 tsp vanilla extract
1/3 cup maltitol
3/4 cup shredded coconut meat, unsweetened
1/4 cup coconut cream, unsweetened
2 tbsps lemon juice
2 cups heavy cream

In large bowl of electric mixer or food processor fitted with steel blade, beat together cream cheese, vanilla extract and maltitol. Beat in coconut, coconut cream (stir well before adding), and lemon juice. In another bowl, whip cream until it forms soft peaks. Fold into cream cheese mixture. Divide mixture among 8 dessert cups. Refrigerate at least 1 hour before serving.

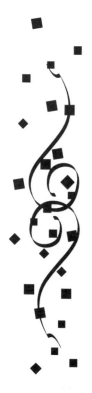

Custard

Serving Size: 6

3 egg yolks
1 egg
1/4 cup maltitol
1 cup heavy cream
1 cup milk
1/2 each vanilla bean
1/4 tsp ground nutmeg

Preheat oven to 325°F. Beat together egg yolks and whole egg until light. Beat in maltitol. Combine vanilla bean, cream and milk, scald, and beat gradually into egg mixture. Scrape vanilla beans into mixture. Pour into six individual custard cups. Sprinkle with freshly grated nutmeg. Place in baking pan and add hot water to reach halfway up sides of cups. Bake for one hour or until a knife inserted into custard comes clean. Serve hot, warm, or cold.

Notes: To make coconut custard, increase the maltitol to 1/3 cup and add 1 cup shredded coconut that is unsweetened.

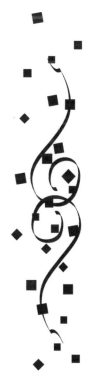

Frozen Chocolate Mousse

Serving Size: 8

1 cup milk
2 ounces unsweetened chocolate
3/4 cup maltitol
1 tsp unflavored gelatin
1 tsp vanilla extract
1 pint heavy cream, whipped

In top of double boiler cook the milk, chocolate, maltitol, and gelatin. Stir frequently. When chocolate is melted and all is combined, beat with whisk until smooth and well blended. Chill until thick, then add vanilla and beat until light. Whip the cream until soft peaks form, then fold gently into chocolate mixture. Place in shallow pan and freeze until firm.

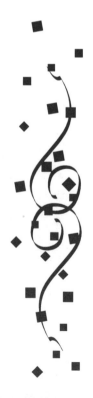

Frozen Coffee Parfait

Serving Size: 4

2 tbsps instant coffee powder
1 tbsp boiling water
6 egg yolks
3/4 cup maltitol
3 tbsps coffee liqueur
2 cups whipping cream

Dissolve coffee powder in water, set aside. In a medium bowl, combine egg yolks and maltitol and beat until foamy, then add to it coffee mixture and liqueur. Beat cream until stiff peaks form, take out one cup and fold the rest into the coffee mixture. Spoon the parfait into cups and freeze until firm. Before serving, spoon reserved whipped cream onto tops of parfaits.

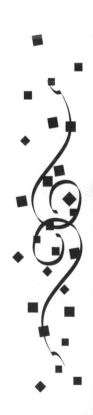

Indian Pudding

Serving Size: 8

2 eggs
6 cups milk
1/2 cup maltitol, honey flavored
1/4 cup brown sugar replacement
1/2 tsp salt
1 tsp cinnamon
1/2 tsp ground ginger
1 cup yellow cornmeal
1/4 cup butter

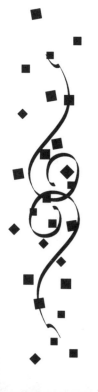

Preheat oven to 325°F and spray a 2 quart baking dish with nonstick cooking spray. In top of double boiler set over hot water, beat together eggs and four cups milk. Beat in maltitol, brown sugar replacement, salt, cinnamon, and ginger and cook until sugar dissolves. Add cornmeal and butter and cook 20 minutes, stirring occasionally. Remove from heat, stir in remaining milk and pour into baking dish. Bake for 3 hours, or until pudding is firm.

Notes: You may add one cup of raisins before baking, if you wish.

Lemon Pear Pudding

Serving Size: 6

3 large pears, peeled & sliced thin
1/4 cup fresh lemon juice
1/3 cup maltitol
1 cup self-rising flour
2/3 cup brown sugar replacement
1 tsp grated lemon zest
1/2 cup margarine

Preheat oven to 400°F and spray an 8 inch square baking dish
with nonstick cooking spray. Combine the first three
ingredients and place them in the prepared baking dish.
Combine the flour, brown sugar substitute and lemon rind
then cut in the margarine with a pastry blender until the
mixture is crumbly. Sprinkle evenly over the pear mixture.
Bake for about 30 minutes, or until golden. Serve warm with
creme fraiche or whipped cream.

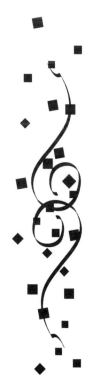

Lowfat Banana Custard

Serving Size: 8

1 cup skim milk
1 whole egg
2 egg yolks
3 tbsps maltitol, maple flavored
3 tbsps all-purpose flour
1 tsp vanilla extract
1 tbsp cornstarch
1 tbsp cold water
2 large bananas

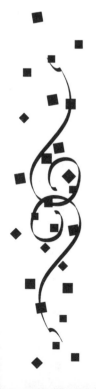

In a small saucepan over medium-high heat, heat milk until it steams. Remove from heat and pour into a mixing bowl. In a separate bowl whisk together egg, egg yolks, and maltitol until smooth. Add flour and vanilla. Mix arrowroot with cold water until it is dissolved and add to egg mixture. Add hot milk. Puree bananas in a blender, then add to egg mixture. Return custard to pan and cook over medium-high heat, stirring, until thick. Pour into 8 dessert glasses and chill in the refrigerator for 4 hours before serving.

Orange Cream Baskets

Serving Size: 6

3 large navel oranges
1/4 cup cold water
1 envelope unflavored gelatin
1 tbsp fresh lemon juice
3 eggs, separated
1/2 cup maltitol
1/4 cup warm water
1/2 cup whipping cream

Cut oranges in half and press out juice (reserve 2/3 cup of juice) making sure to keep the oranges shape. Scrape out the pulp inside the oranges and set the orange shells aside. Pour cold water into a small saucepan and sprinkle gelatin over the top. Let mixture sit for 5 minutes then heat it over low heat to dissolve the gelatin (do not boil). Stir into the gelatin mixture the reserved orange juice and the lemon juice, set aside to cool. Combine egg yolks, maltitol and warm water and beat until foamy. Gradually beat in cooled gelatin mixture and beat until light and fluffy. Refrigerate to firm up some, about 45 minutes. Whip the cream until stiff peaks form and fold it into gelatin mixture. Beat egg whites until stiff and fold them into the gelatin mixture also. Spoon mixture into the reserved orange shells and refrigerate until set, about 2 hours.

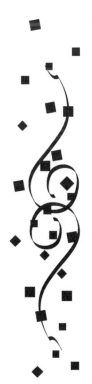

Pumpkin Pudding

Serving Size: 8

1 1/4 cups half and half
1 tbsp cornstarch
1 cup pumpkin puree
2 tbsps cinnamon
1/8 tsp ground cloves
1 tsp ground cardamom
1/2 tsp ground ginger
1/2 tsp nutmeg
3/4 cup maltitol, maple flavored
2 tbsps grated orange rind
2 eggs

Preheat oven to 350°F. Lightly spray 8 custard cups with nonstick cooking spray. In a large bowl combine milk, cornstarch, and molasses, and whisk until well blended. Add pumpkin, cinnamon, cloves, cardamom, gingerroot, nutmeg, maltitol and orange rind. Separate eggs. Add yolks to pumpkin mixture. In a small bowl beat egg whites until stiff peaks form. Fold into pumpkin mixture. Pour into prepared custard cups. Place in a shallow baking pan. Add hot water to one half the height of pan. Bake until firm, about 40 minutes. Let cool slightly before serving or serve chilled.

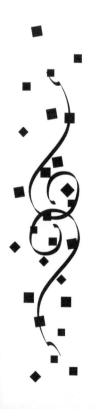

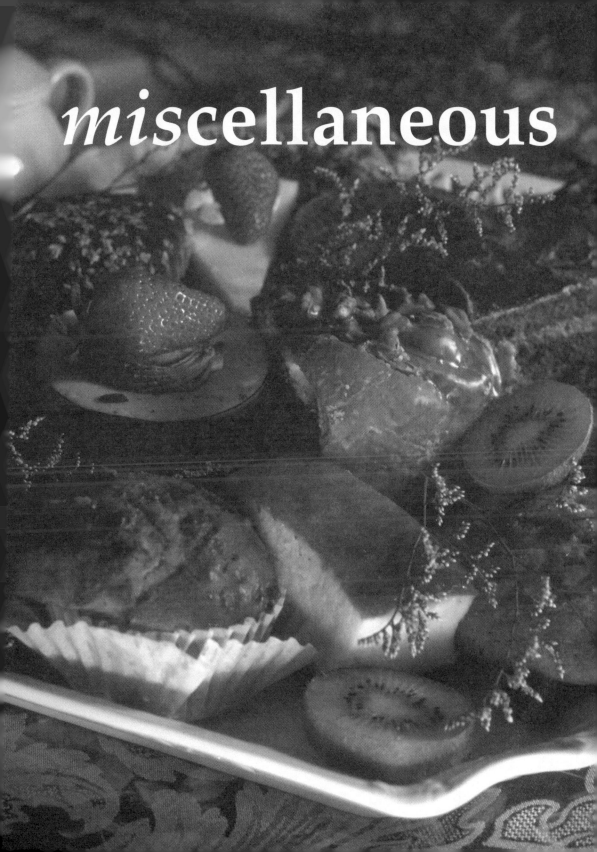

miscellaneous

Pastry Cream

Serving Size: 6

1 cup half and half
1 1/2 tbsps cornstarch
1/8 tsp salt
2 egg yolks, beaten
2 tsps vanilla extract (or 1 vanilla bean)
3 1/2 tsps Equal® sweetener (12 packets)

Combine half and half, cornstarch and salt in a heavy bottomed saucepan and bring to a boil, stirring constantly. Add 1/2 cup of hot mixture to the yolks, then return the mixture to the pot, and turn heat to low. Cook for about 5 minutes until the mixture is very thick. Remove from the heat and add vanilla. Let cream cool for 15 minutes, stirring often to prevent a skin from forming, then stir in Equal. Refrigerate, then allow mixture to cool completely before using.

Notes: To keep a skin from forming on creams and puddings, take a small piece of butter and rub it over the top of the mixture.

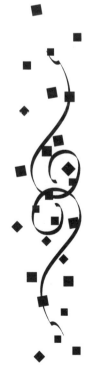

Sweetened Whipped Cream

Serving Size: 8

1 cup heavy cream
3/4 tsp Equal® sweetener
2 tbsps nonfat dry milk powder
1 1/2 tsps vanilla extract

Place cream in a chilled bowl and whip with either a whisk or a mixer. After whipping one minute, sprinkle Equal and dry milk over the cream, and add vanilla. Continue to whip until soft peaks form. Do not overwhip or cream will take on a buttery texture.

Notes: This recipe can be used to frost cakes, top pies, fill cream puffs, or as a garnish on any dessert.

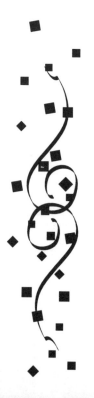

Chocolate Tart Dough

Serving Size: 8

8 tbsps unsalted butter, softened
1/4 cup maltitol
1 tsp vanilla extract
1 egg yolk at room temperature
1/4 cup unsweetened cocoa powder
1 cup all-purpose flour

Place softened butter in a mixing bowl and whip for a couple of minutes or until the butter is fluffy and white. While whipping, add maltitol in a stream and mix until incorporated. Add vanilla extract and egg yolk and mix until well combined. Stop mixing the dough and sift all the cocoa and flour over the mixture, then mix again until no specks of cocoa or flour are visible, about one minute. Form the dough into a ball and place it on a large square of plastic wrap. Place another piece of plastic wrap over it and pat the dough into a 6-8 inch disk. Refrigerate the dough for at least an hour to allow it firm up a little. When you are ready to use the dough, roll it out between the layers of plastic to desired thickness (about 1/8 of an inch for most tarts). When the dough is the correct thickness, peel off the top layer of plastic and place the dough over the tart pan. Push the dough into the pan (dough side down, plastic side up) a little, then peel off the other piece of plastic, and finish pressing the dough into the pan. If the recipe calls for a baked tart crust, pierce the dough with a fork MANY times all over the bottom and sides, then place the pan in an oven preheated to 325°F. Bake for 20-25 minutes, or until the crust is firm. Allow the crust to cool before adding a filling.

Notes: Be sure to sift the flour and cocoa over the mixture because cocoa is very lumpy and doesn't mix in well unless sifted.

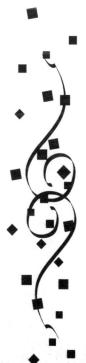

Nutty Tart Crust

Serving Size: 1

1 stick unsalted butter, softened
1/4 cup maltitol
1 tsp vanilla extract
1 egg yolk at room temperature
1/2 cup nuts, ground very fine
1 1/4 cups all-purpose flour

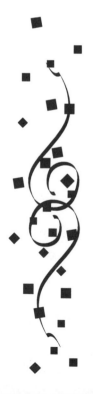

Place softened butter in a mixing bowl and whip for a couple
of minutes or until the butter is fluffy and white. While
whipping, add maltitol in a stream and mix until
incorporated. Add vanilla extract and egg yolk and mix until
well combined. Add nuts and combine. Stop mixing the
dough and sift all the flour over the mixture, then mix again
until no specks of flour are visible, about one minute. Form
the dough into a ball and place it on a large square of plastic
wrap. Place another piece of plastic wrap over it and pat the
dough into a 6-8 inch disk. Refrigerate the dough for at least
an hour to allow it firm up a little. When you are ready to use
the dough, roll it out between the layers of plastic to desired
thickness (about 1/8 of an inch for most tarts). When the
dough is the correct thickness, peel off the top layer of plastic
and place the dough over the tart pan. Push the dough into
the pan (dough side down, plastic side up) a little, then peel
off the other piece of plastic, and finish pressing the dough
into the pan. If the recipe calls for a baked tart crust, pierce the
dough with a fork MANY times all over the bottom and sides,
then place the pan in an oven preheated to 325°F. Bake for 20-
25 minutes, or until the crust is golden. Allow the crust to cool
before adding a filling.

Notes: Two very good nuts to use in this crust are almonds or
hazelnuts. Pecans give the crust an added richness, but
no matter which kind you use, make sure they are
ground finely, almost to a flour.

Pie Crust for a Double-Crusted Pie

Serving Size: 8

2 1/2 cups all-purpose flour
1/2 tsp salt
3/4 cup shortening
6 tbsps cold water

Combine flour and salt, then cut in shortening with a pastry blender or two knives until the mixture looks like coarse cornmeal. Add water, one tablespoon at a time, while mixing with a fork until enough water is added so that the mixture will form a ball. At this point, the dough is ready to be rolled out to be used in another recipe.

Notes: One or two more tablespoons of water may be needed to make the pie dough hold together. Add them one at a time until the right consistency is found.

Quick Hints
Rolling out Sticky Dough
Slip a clean, knee-high stocking over your rolling pen, dust with a little flour and watch sticky dough on the rolling pen disappear!

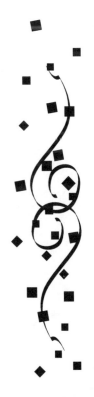

Pie Crust for Single Crust

Serving Size: 8

1 1/2 cups all-purpose flour
1/4 tsp salt
1/2 cup shortening
3 tbsps cold water

Combine flour and salt, then cut in shortening with a pastry blender or two knives until the mixture looks like coarse cornmeal. Add water, one tablespoon at a time, while mixing with a fork until enough water is added so that the mixture will form a ball. At this point, the dough is ready to be rolled out to be used in another recipe.

To bake a pie crust for recipes that call for a pre-baked pie crust, Roll out dough and line a 9 inch pie pan with it. Prick the dough all over the sides and bottom with a fork, and trim off excess dough that hangs over edges. Bake at 425°F for about 16 minutes, or until a light golden brown. Allow crust to cool before filling.

Notes: One or two more tablespoons of water may be needed to make the dough hold together, add then one at a time until it is the right consistency.

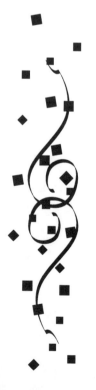

Sweet Tart Dough

Serving Size: 8

1 stick unsalted butter, softened
1/4 cup maltitol
1 tsp vanilla extract
1 egg yolk at room temperature
1 1/4 cups all-purpose flour

Place softened butter in a mixing bowl and whip for a couple of minutes or until the butter is fluffy and white. While whipping, add maltitol in a stream and mix until incorporated. Add vanilla extract and egg yolk and mix until well combined. Stop mixing the dough and sift all the flour over the mixture, then mix again until no specks of flour are visible, about one minute. Form the dough into a ball and place it on a large square of plastic wrap. Place another piece of plastic wrap over it and pat the dough into a 6-8 inch disk. Refrigerate the dough for at least an hour to allow it firm up a little. When you are ready to use the dough, roll it out between the layers of plastic to desired thickness (about 1/8 of an inch for most tarts). When the dough is the correct thickness, peel off the top layer of plastic and place the dough over the tart pan. Push the dough into the pan (dough side down, plastic side up) a little, then peel off the other piece of plastic, and finish pressing the dough into the pan. If the recipe calls for a baked tart crust, pierce the dough with a fork MANY times all over the bottom and sides, then place the pan in an oven preheated to 325°F. Bake for 20-25 minutes, or until the crust is golden. Allow the crust to cool before adding a filling.

Notes: This crust can be rolled out like other pie crusts, but because it tears easily and the high butter content causes it to stick to the table, I find it easier to roll it out between two pieces of plastic.

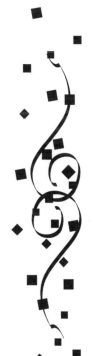

7 Minute Frosting

Serving Size: 10

1 1/2 cups maltitol
1/3 cup cold water
2 egg whites
1/4 tsp cream of tartar
1 tsp vanilla extract

Combine all ingredients except vanilla in the top of a double boiler (the water should be simmering, but not touching the bowl). Beat with an electric mixer on low speed for 30 seconds. Turn the mixer to high and beat for about 7 minutes, or until stiff peaks form. Remove from heat and add vanilla. Beat 2-3 minutes more or until the frosting is spreadable.

Apricot Glaze

Serving Size: 8

3 tbsps apricot preserves, no sugar added
2 tbsps water

Place the preserves and water in a small saucepan. Heat over medium high heat until preserves are melted. Strain if necessary. Brush onto the top of tart, then refrigerate tart to harden glaze.

Notes: It is best to glaze fruit tarts to keep the fruit moist and to give a shiny appearance.

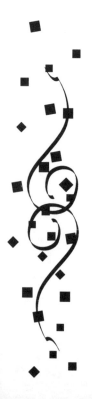

Banana Buttercream

Serving Size: 10

4 large egg whites
1 cup maltitol
3/4 pound unsalted butter, softened
3 tbsps creme de banana or 1 1/2 tsps banana extract

Combine the egg whites and maltitol in a heatproof bowl over a saucepan of simmering water. Whisk the mixture slowly, but constantly until the temperature reaches 140°F, about 4-5 minutes. Remove from heat and whip with a mixer until the meringue is fluffy and at room temperature. While mixing, add the butter a little piece at a time and beat until the buttercream is spreadable. Add banana flavoring and beat 1-2 more minutes. Use immediately.

Chocolate Pudding Frosting

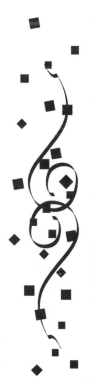

Serving Size: 10

3 tbsps cornstarch
1 cup skim milk
3 ounces unsweetened chocolate squares, chopped fine
1 dash salt
8 tsps Equal® sweetener (25 packets)
2 tbsps butter
1 1/2 tsps vanilla extract

In a heavy saucepan, dissolve cornstarch in milk, then add chocolate and salt and cook over medium heat, stirring constantly, until mixture comes to a boil. Boil one minute, then remove from heat and stir in butter and vanilla. Let cool for 15 minutes, then stir in Equal until it is dissolved. Cover and refrigerate until completely cooled.

Coconut Pecan Frosting

Serving Size: 10

1 egg
5 ounces evaporated milk, not condensed milk
2/3 cup maltitol
1/4 cup unsalted butter
1 1/3 cups unsweetened shredded coconut
1/2 cup chopped pecans

In a heavy saucepan, combine egg, milk and maltitol. Cook over medium heat until very thick, stirring constantly (this will take about 10-15 minutes). Remove from heat and stir in coconut and pecans. Cool frosting completely before frosting a cake with it (you can put it in the refrigerator to speed the cooling process).

Notes: This is the frosting that makes German chocolate cake so yummy!

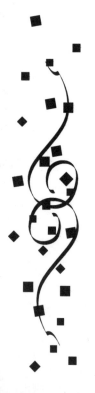

Coffee Buttercream

Serving Size: 10

4 large egg whites
1 cup maltitol
3/4 pound unsalted butter, softened
3 tbsps instant coffee
2 tbsps water

Combine the egg whites and maltitol in a heatproof bowl over a saucepan of simmering water. Whisk the mixture slowly, but constantly until the temperature reaches 140°F, about 4-5 minutes. Remove from heat and whip with a mixer until the meringue is fluffy and at room temperature. While mixing, add the butter a little piece at a time and beat until the buttercream is spreadable. Dissolve the instant coffee in the water and add to the buttercream and whip for 1-2 more minutes. Use immediately.

Cream Cheese Frosting

Serving Size: 10

12 ounces lowfat cream cheese
1/4 cup butter, softened
10 tsps Equal® sweetener
1 tbsp fresh lemon juice
1 tsp vanilla extract

Combine all ingredients in a bowl and whip until all lumps are gone and frosting is fluffy. If mixture gets too warm and starts to melt, refrigerate until firm and whip again.

Notes: This recipe can be made with fat-free cream cheese, but the consistency changes to a thin, glaze-like frosting.

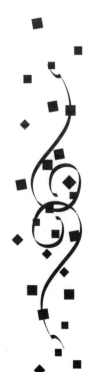

Creme de Menthe Frosting

Serving Size: 10

4 large egg whites
1 cup maltitol
3/4 cup unsalted butter, softened
3 tbsps creme de menthe

Combine the egg whites and maltitol in a heatproof bowl over a saucepan of simmering water. Whisk the mixture slowly, but constantly until the temperature reaches 140°F, about 4-5 minutes. Remove from heat and whip with a mixer until the meringue is fluffy and at room temperature. While mixing, add the butter a little piece at a time and beat until the buttercream is spreadable. Add creme de menthe and whip for 1-2 more minutes. Use immediately.

Ganache

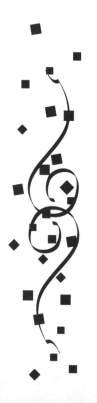

Serving Size: 10

1 cup heavy cream
3/4 cup maltitol
8 ounces unsweetened chocolate squares
4 tbsps butter

Combine the cream and maltitol in a heavy sauce pan over medium heat and bring to a simmer. Remove from heat and add the chocolate and butter. Stir with a whisk until smooth, strain if necessary. At this point, the ganache can be used to pour over a cake or dessert to give it an even chocolate coating. However, if you would like to use it as a frosting, pour it into a bowl and let it come to room temperature. Before using, beat it for a short time with an electric mixer to lighten it up a little.

Lemon Buttercream

Serving Size: 10

4 large egg whites
1 cup maltitol
3/4 pound unsalted butter, softened
3 tbsps fresh lemon juice or 1 1/2 tsps lemon extract

Combine the egg whites and maltitol in a heatproof bowl over
a saucepan of simmering water. Whisk the mixture slowly, but
constantly until the temperature reaches 140°F, about 4-5
minutes. Remove from heat and whip with a mixer until the
meringue is fluffy and at room temperature. While mixing,
add the butter a little piece at a time and beat until the
buttercream is spreadable. Add the lemon juice or extract and
whip for 1-2 more minutes. Use immediately.

Lemon Filling

Serving Size: 10

2 cups maltitol
1/2 cup butter
3 eggs, well beaten
1/2 cup water
3 lemons

Grate rinds of lemons with a grater or zester. Squeeze the
lemons and strain out seeds; use all the lemon juice in recipe.
Cream the butter and maltitol thoroughly; add the eggs and
mix well. Add the water, lemon juice and grated rind. Cook in
top of double boiler until thick. Chill. Use this lemon butter as
filling for eclairs or cakes.

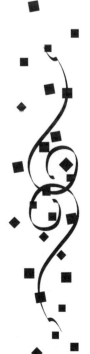

Orange Buttercream

Serving Size: 10

4 large egg whites
1 cup maltitol
3/4 pound unsalted butter, softened
3 tbsps orange juice, frozen concentrate, thawed

Combine the egg whites and maltitol in a heatproof bowl over a saucepan of simmering water. Whisk the mixture slowly, but constantly until the temperature reaches 140°F, about 4-5 minutes. Remove from heat and whip with a mixer until the meringue is fluffy and at room temperature. While mixing, add the butter a little piece at a time and beat until the buttercream is spreadable. Add orange juice concentrate and continue to whip 1-2 more minutes. Use immediately.

Vanilla Buttercream

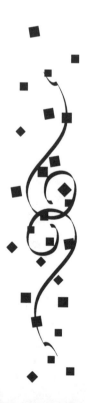

Serving Size: 10

4 large egg whites
1 cup maltitol
3/4 pound unsalted butter, softened
1 tbsp vanilla extract

Combine the egg whites and maltitol in a heatproof bowl over a saucepan of simmering water. Whisk the mixture slowly, but constantly until the temperature reaches 140°F, about 4-5 minutes. Remove from heat and whip with a mixer until the meringue is fluffy and at room temperature. While mixing, add the butter a little piece at a time and beat until the buttercream is spreadable. Add the vanilla extract and whip 1-2 minutes more. Use immediately.

Amaretto Chocolate Sauce

Serving Size: 10

1/2 cup whipping cream
4 ounces unsweetened chocolate, chopped
1/4 cup maltitol
1 tbsp amaretto

Bring cream to a simmer in a small saucepan. Remove from heat. Stir in chocolate until it is melted and mixture is smooth. Stir in maltitol and liqueur.

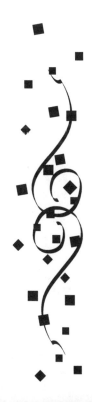

Apricot Sauce

Serving Size: 8

1 1/4 pounds apricots, pitted
1 1/2 cups water
1/3 cup maltitol
1 tbsp cornstarch
1 tbsp cold water

Quarter the apricots and place them in a saucepan with the 1st amount of water and maltitol over medium high heat. Bring the mixture to a boil, then reduce heat to medium and cook about 10-15 minutes, or until the fruit is soft. Pour the contents of the pan into a strainer and push out as much of the fruit pulp as you can with a spatula or spoon. Discard what is left in the strainer and pour the strained mixture back into the saucepan. Combine the cornstarch and the remaining water until all of the cornstarch is dissolved, then add it to the apricot mixture. Bring the sauce to a boil, and boil one minute, stirring constantly. Remove from heat and chill before using. After the mixture has completely cooled, you may add water to the sauce if it is too thick.

Notes: Cornstarch must be dissolved completely in a cold liquid before it is added to a hot liquid for it to thicken properly. If cornstarch is added straight to a hot liquid, it will most likely clump up and not thicken the liquid at all.

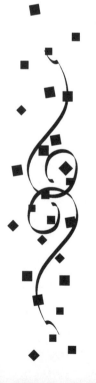

Cassis Sauce

Serving Size: 4

1 pint fresh blackberries
2 tbsps blackberry liqueur
2 tbsps maltitol

Place fruit in food processor or blender. Process until smooth. Press pureed fruit through a sieve into a bowl. Discard seeds left in sieve. Stir liqueur into sauce. Add maltitol, stirring until combined.

Notes: You can use frozen blackberries, but make sure they are unsweetened.

Chocolate Sauce

Serving Size: 8

1 cup water
1 1/3 cups maltitol
2/3 cup unsweetened cocoa powder, sifted
8 ounces unsweetened chocolate (8 1 ounce squares)

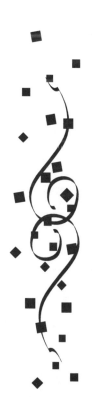

Combine water and maltitol in a saucepan and heat to boiling, then remove from heat. Slowly pour some of the syrup mixture into the cocoa powder until a paste forms. Continue to add the syrup until it is all incorporated into the cocoa powder. Place mixture back on medium heat and cook, stirring occasionally, until the mixture is hot. Remove from heat and add the unsweetened chocolate that has been chopped into small pieces. Stir mixture until sauce is completely smooth. Serve warm or cold.

Notes: Chocolate sauce is much thinner when it is hot, so if you would like to use it cold, you may want to thicken it with a little water to the consistency that you desire.

Cinnamon Sauce

Serving Size: 6

2 tsps cornstarch
1/2 cup cold water
1 1/2 cups boiling water
1 cup brown sugar replacement
1 tsp ground cinnamon
2 tbsps butter
2 tsps vanilla extract

Combine the cornstarch and cold water and stir until the cornstarch is dissolved. Add this mixture to the boiling water bring back to a boil over high heat. Boil, stirring, for one minute. Remove from heat and add remaining ingredients. Serve warm.

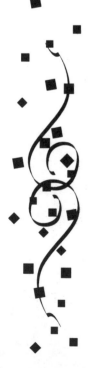

Honey Lemon Sauce

Serving Size: 6

1 cup maltitol, honey flavored
2 tbsps cornstarch
2 cups cold water
1/4 cup unsalted butter
1/4 cup fresh lemon juice
3 tbsps lemon zest, grated

Combine the maltitol and cornstarch in a saucepan. Slowly add the cold water and mix well. Bring mixture to a boil over medium high heat, then add butter, lemon juice and grated lemon peel. Continue to boil slowly until the sauce is thick and opaque, about 3 minutes. Cool slightly before serving or serve chilled.

Hot Fudge Sauce

Serving Size: 8

3/4 cup unsweetened cocoa powder, sifted
1/2 cup brown sugar replacement
1/3 cup maltitol
1/2 cup heavy cream, plus 2 tbsps
1 stick unsalted butter

Combine cocoa powder and brown sugar replacement and set aside. Combine remaining ingredients in a heavy sauce pot over medium high heat and bring to a simmer. Reduce heat to medium and slowly add cocoa mixture to the pot, whisking quickly to avoid lumps. Cook for about 3 minutes more or until the sauce is completely smooth. Serve immediately.

Notes: This sauce must be used hot because it is much too thick for cold use. Store any leftovers covered in the refrigerator, and when you wish to warm it up again, place it in a bowl over simmering water to melt it slowly.

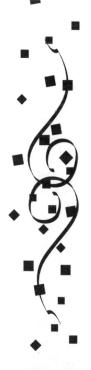

Orange Sauce

Serving Size: 8

2 cups fresh orange juice, strained
2 tbsps cornstarch
1 tbsp fresh lemon juice
1/3 cup maltitol

Mix 1/4 cup of the orange juice with the cornstarch. Combine the remaining ingredients and then add the cornstarch mixture to it. Place all ingredients in a non-reactive saucepan (stainless steel or nonstick coated) and heat to boiling over high heat. Boil for one minute, stirring constantly. Pour sauce into another container, cover and cool completely in the refrigerator. Stir briefly before serving.

Notes: This sauce is surprisingly good spooned over a piece of plain chocolate cake.

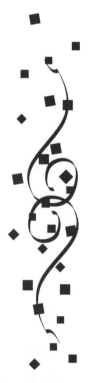

Raspberry Sauce

Serving Size: 8

1 pint fresh raspberries
1/4 cup maltitol or to taste

Combine raspberries and maltitol in a sauce pot over low heat, stirring occasionally. Cook for about 10 - 15 minutes or until raspberries are broken up and hot. Place mixture in a fine strainer, or a double layer of cheesecloth. Press or squeeze out puree to remove seeds and discard seeds. Place sauce, covered, in the refrigerator and serve cold with cake, ice cream or other desserts.

Notes: The tartness of the berries should dictate how much sweetener is added to the sauce. If the berries are very sweet, or you prefer a sauce that is tart, use less sweetener.

appen*dix*

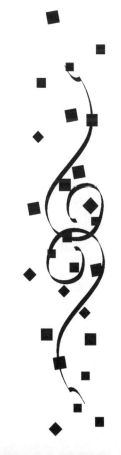

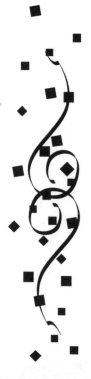

Sugar Terms:

Brown sugar	a soft sugar in which crystals are covered by a refined dark syrup
Carbohydrate	a nutrient made up of sugars and starches
Corn Sugar	a sugar made by the breakdown of cornstarch
Corn Syrup	a containing several types of sugars resulting from the breakdown of cornstarch
Dextrin	a sugar formed by the partial breakdown of starch
Dextrose	another name for sugar
Fructose	a simple sugar found in honey, fruit and juices
Galactose	a simple sugar found in milk sugar or lactose
Glucose	a simple sugar found in blood created by food, and used by the body for heat and energy
Honey	a sweet substance created naturally by bees
Invert Sugar	a sugar combination found in fruit
Lactose	a sugar found in milk
Levulose	another name for fruit sugar
Maltitol	a natural derivative of corn
Maltose	a crystalline sugar formed by the breakdown of starch
Mannitol	a sugar alcohol
Mannose	a sugar derived from manna and the ivory nut
Maple Sugar	a sugar from concentrated sugar maple sap
Molasses	a thick syrup created from raw sugar in the manufacturing of sugar
Sorbitol	a sugar alcohol
Sorghum	a syrup from sorghum grain
Starch	a complex chain of sugars usually found the a powdery form

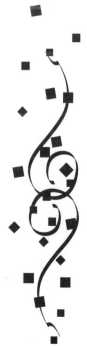

Sucrose	another name for table sugar
Sugar	a carbohydrate, group includes the monosaccharides: fructose, galactose, glucose; and the disaccharides: sucrose, maltose and lactose
Xylose	a wood sugar from in corn cobs, straw, bran woodgum, seed bran, cherries, pears, peaches and plums
Xylitol	a sugar alcohol

Fat List:

Each serving on this list, contains about 5 grams of fat and 45 calories. In your daily intake, you can modify your fat intake by eating unsaturated fats instead of saturated ones.

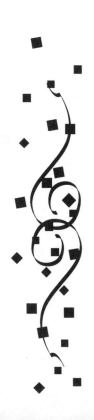

Avocado	1/8 medium
Margarine	1 teaspoon
Margarine, diet**	1 tablespoon
Mayonnaise	1 teaspoon
Mayonnaise, reduced-calorie**	1 tablespoon
Nuts and seeds:	
Almonds, dry roasted	6 whole
Cashews, dry roasted	1 tablespoon
Peanuts	20 small or 10 large
Pecans	2 whole
Walnuts	2 whole
Other nuts	1 tablespoon
Seeds, pine nuts, sunflower (without shells)	1 tablespoon
Pumpkin seeds	2 teaspoons

Oil (corn, cottonseed, safflower, soybean sunflower, olive, peanut)	1 teaspoon
Olives**	10 small or 5 large
Salad dressing, mayonnaise-type	2 teaspoons
Salad dressing, mayonnaise-type, reduced-calorie	1 tablespoon
Salad dressing (oil varieties)**	1 tablespoon
Salad dressing, reduced-calorie	2 tablespoons

Saturated Fats:

Butter	1 teaspoon
Bacon**	1 slice
Chitterlings	1/2 ounce
Coconut, shredded	2 tablespoons
Coffee whitener, liquid	2 tablespoons
Coffee whitener, powder	4 teaspoons
Cream (light, coffee, table)	2 tablespoons
Cream, sour	2 tablespoons
Cream (heavy, whipping)	1 tablespoon
Cream cheese	1 tablespoon
Salt pork**	1/4 ounce

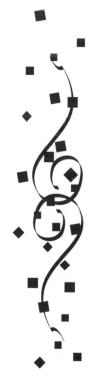

* one serving contains 400 milligrams or more of sodium

** two or more servings provides 400 milligrams or more of sodium

A short note on fat and eggs:
To cut down the fat content in a recipe, eggs are a great place to start! For every whole egg, substitute 2 egg whites. This works great in almost every recipe except muffins, which you need to add 1 extra egg white for every whole egg called for. The only time when the substitution formula doesn't apply is in pies. Pies need the yolks.

Selected Vendors and Suppliers:

Steels's Gourmet Foods
Continental Business Center
Suite D-175
Bridgeport, PA 19405
1-800-6-STEELS
Supplier of maltitol and maltitol-sweetened products

Leroux Creek
970 3100 Road
Hotchkiss, CO 81419
(970) 872-2256
Supplier of unsweetened applesauce and quality food products

Truffle Hound Gourmet, Inc.
1324 Pin Oak Rd.
Katy, TX 77494
(281) 395-2073
Supplier of plain and flavored pastas

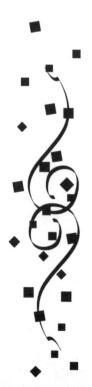

Penzeys, Ltd.
1921 S. West Avenue
Waukesha, WI 53186
(414) 574-0277
Supplier of spices, seasonings and vanilla

Fredericksburg Herb Farm
P.O. Drawer 927
Fredericksburg, TX 78624
(21) 997-8615
Supplier of fresh and dried herbs; herb mixes

Chile Today - Hot Tamale
2-D Great Meadow Lane
East Hanover, NJ 07936
1-800-HOT-PEPPER
Supplier of chili products

index

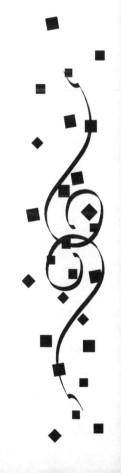